Shamanic Plant Medicine

Ayahuasca:
The Vine of Souls

T0159455

SHAMANIC PLANT MEDICINE

Ayahuasca:
The Vine of Souls

Ross Heaven

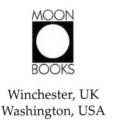

MOON
BOOKS

Winchester, UK
Washington, USA

First published by Moon Books, 2013
Moon Books is an imprint of John Hunt Publishing Ltd., Laurel House, Station Approach,
Alresford, Hants, SO24 9JH, UK
office1@jhpbooks.net
www.johnhuntpublishing.com
www.moon-books.net

For distributor details and how to order please visit the 'Ordering' section on our website.

Text copyright: Ross Heaven 2013

ISBN: 978 1 78279 249 9

A CIP catalogue record for this book is available from the British Library.

Design: Stuart Davies

Printed and bound by CPI Group (UK) Ltd, Croydon, CR0 4YY

We operate a distinctive and ethical publishing philosophy in all
areas of our business, from our global network of authors to
production and worldwide distribution.

CONTENTS

To Bodge, who dreamed this one because she asked for it, and to my kids and Indie.

About the Author

Ross Heaven is the author of several books on shamanism, plant teachers and healing and runs workshops on these themes in Europe and Peru, including Shamanic Practitioner training programmes; Shamanic Healing and Soul Retrieval courses; plant medicine retreats with San Pedro, Salvia and ayahuasca, and journeys to Peru to work with indigenous shamans. He is also a shamanic healer and therapist and offers counselling, soul retrieval and healing in the UK.

He has a website at www.thefourgates.org, where you can read more about his work as well as forthcoming books and other items of interest. He also provides a monthly newsletter by e-mail, which you can receive free of charge by emailing ross@thefourgates.org.

His other books on plant teachers and medicines include *Cactus of Mystery*, *The Hummingbird's Journey to God* and *Drinking the Four Winds* (about San Pedro), *Plant Spirit Shamanism* (about ayahuasca and Amazonian plant healing) and *The Sin Eater's Last Confessions* (about Celtic methods of soul healing with herbs and plants). Others in the Shamanic Plant Medicine series include *Ayahuasca*, *San Pedro* and *Sacred Mushrooms*. His full book list can be viewed at Amazon Books.

Shamanic Plant Medicine
The first practical guide to working with teacher plants

Shamanic Plant Medicine is a series of books written to provide you with a succinct and practical introduction to a specific *teacher* or *power plant*, its history, shamanic uses, healing applications and benefits, as well as the things to be aware of when working with these plants, including ceremonial procedures and safety precautions. These plants are also known in the Western world as *entheogens*: substances which 'reveal the God within', and in shamanic cultures as *allies*: helpful spirits which confer power and pass on insights and information.

The first in this series are *Ayahuasca: The Vine of Souls, San Pedro: The Gateway to Wisdom, Salvia Divinorum: The Sage of the Seers* and *Sacred Mushrooms: Messengers of the Stars*. It is a series which reveals the truth about these plants and provides an insight into their uses as well as the cautions to take with them, so you are properly informed of your choices not reliant on sensationalism and disinformation.

The shamanic use of plants and herbs is one of the world's oldest healing methods and, despite propaganda to the contrary, it is usually the safest and most effective form of medicine too.

In 2005 for example the British Medical Journal warned that, 'in England alone reactions to drugs that led to hospitalisation followed by death are estimated at 5,700 a year and could actually be closer to 10,000'. By comparison, between 2000 and August 2004 there were just 451 reports of adverse reactions to herbal preparations and only 152 were considered serious. No fatalities. That statistic equates to just 38 problem cases a year resulting from plant medicines compared to perhaps 10,000 deaths a year as a result of accepted mainstream medicine. Reviewing these figures the London Independent newspaper concluded that, 'Herbs may not be completely safe as critics like to point out – but they are a lot safer than drugs.'

The situation in America is very similar. Here, orthodox medical treatment itself is now the leading cause of death, ahead of heart disease and cancer, and, 'Infections, surgical mistakes and other medical harm contributes to the deaths of 180,000 hospital patients a year [and] another 1.4 million are seriously hurt by their hospital care.' (Consumer Reports online: www.consumerreports.org). Other studies reveal that adverse drug reactions are under-reported by up to 94 per cent since the US government does not adequately track them. Death as a result of plant healings meanwhile remain next to zero.

It is worth asking why these figures so often go unreported, and why the medical profession continues to treat people as it does, even with full awareness of the risks and comparisons. Another good question would be why plants and herbs more than drugs and orthodox medicine are the focus of governments for stricter regulation (see for example the current *codex alimentarius* proposals) despite their effectiveness and comparative freedom from risk. Who benefits?

More remarkable even than their ability to heal the body is the ability of some plants to expand the mind, raise consciousness, release stuck or damaging emotions and connect us more deeply to spirit. These are the teacher plants. By showing us our true power and potential they enable us to see through illusions and explore the real nature of the dreaming universe so we discover our purpose on Earth.

Plant teachers are used by shamans the world over in a sacred ritual context to divine the future, enter spirit realms, learn the deepest truths of themselves and the universe (although many shamans see little distinction between the two since, as they say, 'the world is as you dream it'; that is, each of us *is* the universe).

They also enable them – and us – to perform *true* healings which go beyond the abilities of modern medicine and its reliance on intrusive treatments and often damaging drugs.

Ayahuasca: The Vine of Souls

The ayahuasca landscape is a virtual battleground populated with malevolent spirits but also with allies, plant teachers, animal spirit guides, ancestral spirits and other morally ambiguous entities. The shaman's task is essentially one of extra-dimensional diplomacy; that is, to identify and forge alliances with the beneficial entities while guarding against those that don't necessarily have one's best interests in mind.

Dennis McKenna, *The Brotherhood of the Screaming Abyss*

1

The Vine of Souls and the Amazonian Approach to Healing

My experience was nothing short of life-changing. I was led into a new world where darkness and fear is transformed into love and light. My ceremonies showed me far more than I thought possible and have given me a true understanding of what is necessary to return to my natural state. I purged years of physical pains, fears and cultural programming from my mind, body and spirit. I also received downloads of spiritual knowledge and instructions on how to remain connected to god/nature.
Shane, Australia[1]

Ayahuasca – a simple Amazonian vine – has, in the past few decades, spread its tendrils from the remote forests where it grows to destinations worldwide and has come to be seen by some of those who have drunk it (a varied bunch including musicians, models, doctors, lawyers, nurses, actors, artists, tradespeople, businessmen and women, to mention just some of those who have attended my workshops with the plant) as a sort of panacea for our age; a 'living God' which can put us back in touch with our souls and lead to new understanding and the potential for a peaceful Earth.

The vine seems now to be everywhere – almost an 'overnight sensation' – known to Western shamans far removed from the Amazon rainforests, and to non-healers alike. Even the mainstream media is aware of it and, while it would normally fly into a moral outrage about the brew (as it does with all 'drugs', calling for them to be banned as soon as it is aware of them), it has until now at least taken a more restrained and considered view about ayahuasca, perhaps partly due to the positive words that have been spoken about it by celebrities and musicians including Sting, Tori Amos, Paul Simon and even the fresh-faced and wholesome Olivia Newton John.

Every leaf, every blade of grass, every nodding flower is reaching out, every insect calling to me, every star in the clear sky sending a direct beam of light to the top of my head. This sensation of connectedness is overwhelming. It's like floating in a buoyant limitless ocean of feeling that I can't really begin to describe unless I evoke the word love. Before this experience I would have used the word to separate what I love from everything I don't love – us not them, heroes from villains, friend from foe, everything in life separated and distinct like walled cities or hilltop fortresses jealously guarding their hoard of separateness. Now all is swamped in this tidal wave of energy which grounds the skies to the earth so that every article of matter in and around me is vibrant with significance. Everything around me seems in a state of grace and eternal.

Sting (in his autobiography, *Broken Music*)

It was one of the most influential journeys I have ever had being in ceremony with ayahuasca, the vine from the Amazon... It's very much a journey that a real medicine woman [or]medicine man has to take you on, where you go inside. It's not a social thing and it's not something you should do on your own. It's an internal experience... And yes, it does sometimes give me visions. But my intention when I am doing it is very different than recreational. I don't do it recreationally. I do it to go do inner work.

Tori Amos

[My album] 'Spirit Voices' is really based on events that happened to me on a trip into the Amazon. We went to see a shaman in a shack in a jungle... first he sang. He sang for a long

time, chanted... these beautiful melodies... and then they made up this brew called ayahuasca... which we drank.
Paul Simon

I have realized the ritual of ayahuasca in Pucallpa and I have shared a few days with the Shipibo, whose members are wonderful people... Peru is a charming land.
Olivia Newton John

Cut to February 2012 and the mega-celebrity, Jennifer Aniston, best known for playing perky girl-next-door Rachel in *Friends*, is tipping a bowl of ayahuasca to her lips in Universal's newest romantic comedy *Wanderlust*. In just a few years, the once secret 'shaman's brew' of the Amazon has snaked its way into the popular consciousness, including the entertainment industry, with cameos in the TV shows *Weeds* and *Nip/Tuck* and now the movie *Wanderlust*...

This ancient ayahuasca healing modality has proven effective in cases where Western medicine failed. In *Black Smoke*, author Margaret DeWys describes how 'the spirit vine' cured her of terminal breast cancer... and National Geographic adventurer Kira Salak wrote about how overcoming a 'devil' in an ayahuasca vision vanquished her life-long struggle with depression in what has become 'the most popular article the magazine has ever published, bringing in 20 times more reader response mail than any previous article.'
Jonathan Talat Phillips in The Huffington Post.[2]

Ayahuasca has always been good at making its own mythology so we must be careful about over-claiming the undoubtedly remarkable qualities of this plant and portraying it as something miraculous.[3]

Amazing cures and spiritual illumination are certainly possible from working seriously with it. However, although this normally requires more than one ceremony or one drink of the brew, but a rigorous healing process of which ayahuasca is one important part. (More on this in the section below).

An Introduction to the Vine

The word ayahuasca comes from two native Quechua words: *aya* meaning 'spirit', 'soul, or 'ancestor', and *huasca* meaning 'vine' or 'rope'. Hence it is known as the vine of souls'. It plays a central role in the spiritual and cultural traditions of the Amazon and, in 2008, was constitutionally recognised by the Peruvian government as a National Treasure.

Its ceremonial use dates back thousands of years. One of the earliest objects related to it is a specially-engraved cup, now a museum piece, which was found in the Amazon around 500 BC and shows that ayahuasca has been used as a sacrament for at least 2,500 years.

The brew is made from ayahuasca vine (*Banisteriopsis caapi*) and the leaves of the chacruna plant (*Psychotria viridis*), and it is said that a shaman can find plentiful sources of both by listening for the heartbeat that emanates from them.[4]

The ayahuasca mixture is prepared by adding the vines and leaves to water and boiling it for several hours so that it reduces to a thick brown potion. This is the brew that is drunk. The shaman oversees the entire process, often blowing good intentions for healing and tobacco smoke into the mixture (a procedure known as *soplada*), singing magical chants called *icaros* to it and offering prayers to the ayahuasca spirits for a successful ceremony to follow.

Icaros

Icaros, the sacred songs of the shaman, are integral to the ayahuasca experience and direct the ceremony and the visions which may arise. The shaman has songs for each person's needs, the vibrations of which summon healing energies with words that tell of nature's ability to heal.

For example, an icaro may call in the energy of a sacred stream to wash away illness or of brightly-coloured flowers with the power to attract good fortune. As the shaman sings you might even see these things in your visions (ayahuasca was once known by the scientific name *telepathine* because of its ability to work in this way, suggesting that it engenders a form of telepathy among its drinkers so that they share common thoughts, images or experiences during ceremony).

Icaros may also be used to call protective spirits, summon the essence of nature, and to provoke the *mareacion* or effects of the ayahuasca by making a plea to the spirit of the vine. In the words of one ayahuascero (Javier, quoted in my book, *Plant Spirit Shamanism*), icaros 'render the mind susceptible for visions; then the curtains can open for the start of the theatre'.

Icaros are not always songs per se but may also be magical chants or a melody that is whistled or whispered into the ayahuasca brew or into the energy field of a person who is to be healed during a ceremony. Rather than hymns (which are more common in the Brazilian Santo Daime tradition, a fusion of ayahuasca shamanism and Christianity), Amazonian icaros are better regarded as an energetic force charged with positive healing intent. The shaman stores this force inside his body and is able to transmit it to another person or to the brew itself so that this life-giving energy is also ingested when the mixture is drunk.

These songs are taught to the shaman by the spirit of the plants themselves; the longer his relationship with these plants, the more icaros he may learn and the more potent they will be. The power and knowledge of an ayahuascero is therefore sometimes measured in part by the number of icaros he possesses. Javier, for example, claims to know the spirit songs of some 1,500 'jungle doctors', including the *icaro del tabaco* (the song of tobacco – one of the most sacred of Amazonian plants), the *icaro del ajo sacha* (the song of the plant ajo sacha – see below) and the *icaro del chiric sanango* (also see below), among many others.

However, it is not always true that a library of songs automatically equals greater power since, with the rise of ayahuasca tourism in Peru, there are now a number of 'song and dance' shamans who know plenty of good tunes and are willing to sing them in ceremonies for visitors but who do not themselves have great healing gifts. They are, sadly, more like entertainers. On the other hand, there are also shamans like don Luis of Iquitos who know fewer plants but know them extremely well. His primary ally is chiric sanango, a plant he has dieted many times, the first for a period of 18 months in contrast to the usual shamanic plant diet of just 14 days. In Luis' view it is more important to know a few plants extremely well and to have them as well-established friends and allies because then they will act as your ambassador in the spirit world and lead you to the plants you need for a patient no matter what his illness.

There are precise and specific icaros for many different purposes – to cure snake bites, for example, or to clarify visions during ayahuasca ceremonies, to communicate with the spirit world, or even to win the love of a woman. *Huarami icaros* (from the Quechua word *huarami* which, loosely, means 'woman') are of this latter category. Others – *icaros de las piedras* – are taught to shamans by *encantos* (special healing stones which offer spiritual protection), while *icaros del viento* call upon the spirit of the wind and *ayaruna icaros* (from the Quechua words *aya* – 'spirit' or 'dead' – and *runa* – 'people' – are sung to invoke the 'spirit people' – the souls of dead shamans who live in the underwater world – so they may help during a healing or an ayahuasca ceremony.

Icaros can also be transmitted from a master shaman to his

disciple but it is nature that is regarded as the greatest teacher and the most powerful songs are those learnt directly from plants themselves. To learn these songs the shaman must follow a special diet for many weeks as he treks deep into the rainforest to find the appropriate plants and places of power where the magical music of nature can be heard. The words of the chants he then learns are symbolic stories telling of the ability of nature to heal itself and heal us, since we are a part of nature too. What actually heals, however, is not the words or the tune but the healing vibration they carry and the insights that arise from this, which allow inner feelings to unblock so that bitterness and anger can change to ecstasy and love.

The Shamanic Diet

Ayahuasca is sometimes also called the purge (*la purga*) and has a reputation for causing vomiting. It is worth saying something about this here. Firstly, it is not 'compulsory' that you vomit! Many people do not.

In Peru, however, purging is regarded as beneficial because when people purge the spirit of ayahuasca is conducting a healing. What emerges from the body is often not physical matter at all but unhealthy energies that lead to illness.

During an ayahuasca session, for example, you might make a healing connection between a negative event from your past and a pattern of *saladera* (bad luck) you are experiencing now, followed by an urge to vomit. What comes up is the negative energy from that event so that new, positive energies can flow. This is a purification of the soul so your luck can change for the better and old attachments and limitations are released.

Adherence to a special diet as part of the ayahuasca *process* of healing will also reduce the likelihood of vomiting (as opposed to purging). The diet in fact is a key part of the experience and can be a journey of self-exploration and discovery in itself, bringing greater awareness our routines and habits which can limit us. As Barbara, one of my American participants, put it: 'Judging from people's comments, I think the diet was harder for me than everyone else. This led to the insight of how much of my life is centred around food.'

Shamanic diets also enhance the visionary experience. They involve purification, retreat, commitment and respect for our connection to everything around us. Through the exclusion of some foodstuffs and activities the diet enables us to purify and take in the spirit of ayahuasca and its healing. They are also key to the training of every shaman as he develops his relationship with new plant allies.

As part of the diet – whether undertaken by a shaman to meet a new plant spirit or administered to a patient to heal a particular illness – other (typically non-entheogenic) plants are usually taken, each of which has a specific healing function on a physical and a psycho-spiritual level.

The objective in taking them is not to cure a *symptom* of illness (which is the focus of Western medicine) but to find and release the underlying *cause* by taking in the spiritual power of the plant so that it is always with you and feeding you its strength. This is based on the notion that plants have a personality and intention of their own which is more wide-ranging than their purely physical properties. A plant like manzanilla (chamomile), for example, is known in the West as a relaxant and a stress-reliever and, of course, in Peru it provides this service too but its deeper spiritual personality is concerned with 'lightening the load' or 'smoothing the way'. Once its power is a part of us at the end of a successful diet it can therefore be called upon to relieve stress and make things easier for us not just on a bodily level but, through magic and intention, in all situations we come into contact with.

These are so many other examples of plants that are commonly dieted. Some (known as admixtures) may also be added to the ayahuasca brew to produce particular healing effects.

Jergon Sacha

Jergon is a 'signature plant', its spiritual essence (or ally) advertising its presence and healing intentions through its appearance. The look and colouration of its stem resembles a poisonous snake which is indigenous to the area in which it grows and a medicine made from the root of the plant is the only known antidote to a bite from this snake. The plant is therefore a lifesaver when a root poultice is applied to the bite and an infusion of the tuber in water is drunk. The wider spiritual intention of this plant, shamanically speaking, therefore, is to extract poisons (*virotes*: magical darts of negative energy, sometimes sent by rivals or black magicians) which have attached themselves to us as 'viral infections'. These then manifest in our energy bodies – and eventually our physical bodies – in various forms, such as cancers and other diseases. Jergon sacha removes these energy darts and cleanses the physical and spiritual body. For this reason it has also proven useful in clinical studies in the treatment of addictions, cancer, HIV and AIDS.

Tobacco

Nicotiana rustica, known in South America as *mapacho*, is a potent form of tobacco which is sometimes added to ayahuasca to clarify visions and provoke purging to rid the body of parasites and toxins. The recreational use of tobacco is rare among Amazonian Indians but in ceremonies where ayahuasca is taken it is common for shamans (and participants) to smoke huge cigars, some as long as 36 inches, to purify the ritual space and keep unwanted spirits out. The spirit of tobacco is seen by some shamans as a beautiful woman dressed in white, by others as a black smoke-like shape and by others as the plant itself but in gigantic multi-leaved form and in brilliant colours. Her attitude is motherly, healing and loving but she does demand absolute adherence to the diet and the consequences of breaking it can be severe. It is not therefore a plant to be trifled with since it is both a healer and a destroyer. It may be used by the shaman to cure addictions, pulmonary illnesses, breathing problems and cancers, for example (and in recent medical studies in the West is also showing promise as a treatment for some forms of cancer), but it can also aid spirit extraction work by suffocating, weakening or killing negative entities. The greater ('mother') spirit of the plant also contains other allies with specific functions, such as warriorship (endurance) and healing (cleansing and relaxation).

Ortega

When seen shamanically ortega (nettle) resembles a short snake made of bright green leaves which enters the body of a patient and begins the process of stinging or burning out any intrusive energy it finds. Like jergon sacha, the spiritual intention of the plant is to remove poisons, viruses or entities and to cleanse the physical and spiritual body.

In the West, nettle has been found to reduce allergies, cleanse the blood, relieve pain, lower blood pressure, and can be used as a diuretic and to help cure arthritis, rheumatism, ulcers, asthma, diabetes, and intestinal inflammation, and this is also why it is used in Peru. According to Leslie Taylor in *The Healing Power of Rainforest Herbs*, 'Several of nettle's lectin chemicals have demonstrated marked antiviral actions (against HIV and several common upper respiratory viruses). Other chemicals... have been documented with interesting immune stimulant actions... In one study, a nettle root extract was shown to inhibit the growth of prostate cells by 30 per cent in five days. Another reported it inhibited BPH [Benign Prostatic Hyperplasia] in mice by 51.4 per cent (which suggested it could be used as a preventative as well as a treatment)', which gives credence to the shaman's view of the spiritual intention of this plant.

Pinon Colorado

Pinon is used as a defence against evil sorcerers. 'Evil sorcerers' are around us everywhere, incidentally. Every time we get on the tube and sit next to someone who is radiating hostility because they've had a bad day we expose ourselves to negative vibrations and bad energy. This has a real physical effect – like that sick feeling in the stomach when someone acts or speaks aggressively towards us – and this energy can stick. Pinon colorado is a cure against emanations like these as well as more deliberate attacks by rivals, competitors and black magicians in all walks of life.

Chiric Sanango

Chiric sanango grows mainly in the upper Amazon and in a few *restingas* (high ground which never floods). It is good for colds and arthritis and has the effect of heating up the body. (*Chiric*, in Quechua, means 'tickling' or 'itchy', an allusion to the prickly heat it generates). Shamans often prescribe it for fishermen and loggers, for example, because they spend so much time in the water and are prone to colds and arthritis. The patient should not drink too much at a time though because it can lead to numbness of the mouth as well as a feeling of slight disorientation. It is also used in magical baths (see below) to change the bather's energy and bring good luck to his ventures and is sometimes added to ayahuasca. Its spirit is said to look like a black man, a knight on horseback, dressed in armour and carrying a lance and a sword: a warrior ally whose primary gift is power. It also has a more psychological effect, but still to do with 'heat' since it enables people to open their hearts to love (it 'warms up' a cold heart, but will also 'cool' a heart that is inflamed with jealousy or rage) and to identify with others 'as if they were brothers and sisters'. In essence, it helps people get in touch with a more sensitive and loving part of themselves. Another of its gifts is enhanced self-esteem, which develops from this more healthy connection to the self.

Guayusa

This is a good plant for people who suffer from excessive acidity, digestive, or other problems of the stomach and bile. It also develops mental strength and is paradoxical in the sense that, just as chiric sanango is cooling and warming at the same time, guayusa is both energizing and relaxing. It also has the effect of giving lucid dreams (i.e. when you are aware that you are dreaming and can direct your dreams). For this reason it is sometimes known as the 'night watchman's plant', as even when you are sleeping you have an awareness of your outer surroundings. The boundary between sleeping and wakefulness becomes fluid and dreams become more colourful, richer, and more potent than before.

Ajo Sacha

Ajo is a blood purifier and helps the body rid itself of toxins (spiritual or physical) as well as restoring strength and equilibrium lost through illnesses that have an effect on the blood. Psycho-spiritually, it helps to develop acuity of mind and can also take the user out of *saladera* (a run of bad luck, inertia, or a sense of not living life to the full). It is also used for ridding spells – i.e. undoing the work of curses or removing bad energy that has been sent deliberately or by accident (in an explosion of rage, etc.). Used in floral baths, it will relieve states of shock and fear (known as *manchiari*), which can be particularly debilitating to children, whose souls are not as strong or fixed as an adult's; a powerful shock can therefore lead to soul loss. Another key to ajo sacha is that in the Amazon it is used to enhance hunting skills, not only by covering the human scent with its own garlic-like smell (the plant also has a garlic taste although it is not related to garlic), but by amplifying the hunter's senses of taste, smell, sound, and vision, which are essential for success and survival. It is a plant of stalking and this ability also translates psychologically, enabling an individual to hunt or 'stalk' her inner issues.

The ayahuascero Guillermo adds that it opens up the shamanic path and helps the apprentice see beyond conventional reality – as long as he has 'the heart of a warrior and is prepared to live under the obligations of shamanism. For this, he will need courage, the ability to face the truth, and to know his true calling, without fear of extremes or 'ugly' things'.

Mocura/Mucura

In appearance the ally of mucura is somewhat like the plant itself but in human form: tall and spindly with many arms. Known as a 'sorcerer's plant', its essence is the removal of witchcraft and negative energy and for this reason, again, it has been shown to kill cancerous cells, to prevent tumours, to kill viruses and strengthen the immune response. Mucura was one of just 34 plants (in a study of more than 1,400) identified with active properties against cancer in research conducted at the University of Illinois. In another study the plant was shown to be toxic to leukaemia and lymphoma cancer cells. Other studies demonstrate its toxicity to liver and brain cancer cells. It may also be effective as a treatment for diabetes (a traditional use for the plant in the rainforest): 'Researchers in 1990 demonstrated the in vivo hypoglycaemic effect of [mucura], showing that [it] decreased blood sugar levels by more than 60 per cent one hour after administration to mice.' (Leslie Taylor)

The plant also boosts emotional powers (empathy) and brings equilibrium. For this reason it is regarded as a 'great balancer', restoring the connection between the rational mind and the feeling self. For example, it is good at countering shyness and can enhance one's sense of personal value and authority by helping overcome painful memories (of past embarrassments and 'failures', etc.). It is also used in floral baths to cleanse and protect against malevolent forces such as sorcery and *envidia* (envy).

Rosa Sisa

Rosa sisa (marigold) is often used to heal children who are suffering from *mal aire* ('bad air'), which can occur, for example, when a family member dies and leaves the child unhappy and sleepless. The spirit of the dead person lingers, it is said, because it is sad to go and aware of the grief around it, so it stays in the house and tries to comfort its family. This proximity to death, however, can make children ill. Rosa sisa is also used to bring good luck and harmony in general. One of the ways that bad luck can result is through the magical force of envidia. A jealous neighbour might, for instance, throw a handful of graveyard dirt into your house to spread sadness and heavy feelings. Those in the house become bored, agitated, or restless as a consequence. The solution is to take a bucket of water and crushed rosa sisa flowers and thoroughly wash the floors to dispel the magic. Many Peruvians also grow rosa sisa near the front door of their houses to absorb the negativity of people who pass by and look in enviously to see what possessions they have. The flowers turn black when this happens, but go back to their normal colour when the negative energy is dispersed through the roots of the plant to the Earth.

Piri Piri

Piri piri is used to treat a wide range of health problems. The roots, for example, will cure headaches, fevers, cramps, dysentery and wounds, as well easing childbirth and protecting babies from illness. Since it is used for such a wide range of conditions, its powers were once dismissed as superstition. Pharmacological research, however, reveals the presence of ergot alkaloids within the plant, which are known to have diverse effects on the body – from stimulation of the nervous system to the constriction of blood vessels. These alkaloids are responsible for the wide range of uses, but come, not from the plant itself, but from a fungus that infects it. Special varieties of piri piri are cultivated by Shipibo women to improve their artistic skills, especially in weaving the visionary tapestries the Shipibo are famous for, which are said to embody the spiritual universe. It is customary when a girl is very young for her mother to squeeze a few drops of sap from the piri piri seed into her eyes to give her the ability to have visions of the designs she will make when she is older.

Una de Gato

Una de Gato ('cat's claw') is a vine which gets its name from the small thorns at the base of its leaves, which look like a cat's claw and enable it to wind itself around trees, climbing to a height of up to 150 feet. The inner bark of the vine has been used for generations to treat inflammations, colds, viral infections, arthritis, and tumours. It also has anti-inflammatory and blood-cleansing properties, and will clean out the intestinal tract to treat a wide array of digestive problems such as gastric ulcers, parasites, and dysentery. Its most famous quality, however, is its powerful ability to boost the body's immune system, and it is considered by many shamans to be a 'balancer', returning the body's functions to a healthy equilibrium.

From a psycho-spiritual or shamanic perspective, disease usually arises from a spiritual imbalance within the patient, causing him to become de-spirited or to lose heart (in the West we might call this depression). Interestingly, Thomas Bartram, in his *Encyclopaedia of Herbal Medicine*, writes that in the West, 'some psychiatrists believe [problems of the immune system, where the body attacks itself] to be a self-produced phenomenon due to an unresolved sense of guilt or dislike of self... People who are happy at their home and work usually enjoy a robust immune system.' The psychiatric perspective, in this sense, is not so different from the shamanic view. Cat's claw is believed to heal illness by restoring peace to the spirit as well as the balance between spirit and body. The medicinal properties of this plant are officially recognized by the Peruvian government and it is a protected (for export) plant.

Chullachaqui Caspi

The resin of the chullachaqui caspi tree, extracted from the trunk in the same way as rubber from the rubber tree, can be used as a poultice or smeared directly onto wounds to heal deep cuts and stop haemorrhages. For skin problems, such as psoriasis, the bark can be grated and boiled in water while the patient sits before it, covered with a blanket, to receive a steam bath. The deeper, more spiritual, purpose of this tree is to help the shaman or his patient get close to the spirit of the forest and in touch with the vibration and rhythm of the Earth. This reconnection with nature will strengthen an unsettled mind and help to ground a person who is disturbed. It will also guide and protect the apprentice shaman and show him how to recognise which plants can heal.

The tree has large buttress roots as it grows in sandy soil where roots cannot penetrate deeply (*chulla* in Quechua means 'twisted foot' and *chaqui* means plant). This forms part of Amazonian mythology, in stories of the jungle 'dwarf', the *chullachaqui*, which is said to have a human appearance, with one exception: his twisted foot. The chullachaqui is the protector of the forest, and lives in places where the tree also grows. The legend is that if you are lost in the forest and meet a friend or family member, it is most likely the chullachaqui who has taken their form. He will be friendly and suggest going for a walk so he can guide you or show you something of interest. If you go, however, he will lead you deeper into the jungle until you are lost, and you will then suffer madness or become a chullachaqui yourself. Perhaps this legend refers to the initiation of plant shamans, who must also go into the jungle to pursue their craft by getting to know the plants and the forest, taking them away from 'normal society' and therefore into a form of 'madness'. It must be said, however, that Amazonian shamans believe literally in the existence of the chullachaqui; many claim to have met him. At least one, Javier, says he has a photograph of the jungle dwarf to prove it (although, in fairness, he has never shown it to me and I have asked many times!)

Chuchuhuasi

This is another Amazonian tree which forms an important part of the jungle pharmacopoeia. The bark can be chewed as a remedy for stomach ache, fevers, arthritis, circulation issues, and bronchial problems, but it is rather bitter and so more often it is boiled in water and honey. Chuchuhuasi is also regarded as a 'libido stimulant' and aphrodisiac, giving the person who drinks it a renewed sense of life and vigour and this, then, is its spiritual intention: to create passion, to stimulate creativity and, ultimately, to bring us love.

Brugmansia

Brugmansia, *toe*, or *datura* is an extremely potent visionary plant. The entire plant is psychoactive and from ingestion of just a few leaves or flowers a trance results – described by many shamans as a form of madness – which can last for days. Some shamans choose to undergo this ordeal, however, as it is said that the plant gives them the ultimate power of life and death. In the right hands, then, brugmansia can be an exceptional healer. It is nevertheless more often associated with sorcery and black magic (*brujeria*).

It is sometimes (although less so these days) added to ayahuasca as an admixture. I have drunk it many times in this way and it certainly enhances the visionary experience although the information it provides is often negative in nature (showing you all your wrongs, like a nagging, persistent mother) and the images it provides can be too fast-moving to really make sense of. Some writers go even further and offer a warning against the plant, such as Dennis McKenna in *The Brotherhood of the*

Screaming Abyss: 'I've had ayahuasca laced with *toe* (the traditional name for Brugmansia) and it doesn't enhance the experience. One can often tell the additive is present in the ayahuasca brew because the tropanes [it contains] cause a 'dry mouth' effect, inducing a persistent severe thirst which is part of their anti-cholinergic effect. If you should ingest ayahuasca that induces this effect there is a good chance that it contains *toe* as an admixture and *that*, in turn, is a good sign that you are dealing with a brujo, a witch, and a person of dubious character.' I wouldn't go quite that far but I would agree that brugmansia is not a plant to take lightly and a lot of caution should be used when working with it.

Other rainforest plants

There are, of course, thousands of plants in the rainforest (Leslie Taylor remarks, in *The Healing Power of Rainforest Herbs*, that 'Around 125,000 species – almost half the plants on Earth – are found in tropical rainforests [and]... There is no doubt that many of these plants hold the keys to life-saving new medicines – we know this from the less-than-one-per cent that have been studied.') So, the list above is far from exhaustive.

What is common to all of them, however, is that dieting any plant is radically different to taking a pharmaceutical. The latter has an effect only on the body and only while the course of drugs continues, whereas plant medicines lead to a permanent change through the relationship you establish with the spirit of the plant itself. This is the purpose of dieting in fact: to create a connection of power, and why the diet is almost always part of an ayahuasca-based healing treatment. Ayahuasca opens us up to the spirit of the plants, but it is often these other plants rather than the vine per se which provide the healing. It is also why stories of 'miracle cures' from a single drink of ayahuasca should be treated with caution. It *is* possible, but more typically ayahuasca healing is a *process* which involves other elements such as the energy medicine of the icaros, the use of other plants, and cleansing baths or *banos florales* ('flower baths').

Cleansing Baths

Herbal and floral baths use specially chosen plants and flowers with particular spiritual effects for purification and empowerment. Flowers, leaves or roots are added to cooling river water and the mixture is poured over the body as a blessing to restore balance and harmony to the soul, washing away unhelpful spirits so that blockages are removed and the energy of the universe can flood in to correct the imbalance. By cleansing and 'flourishing' us they also prepare us for the deeper healing of ayahuasca.

Shipibo shaman, Artidoro, describes the process in my book *Plant Spirit Shamanism*.

The bath is most often taken on the morning after ayahuasca ceremonies so that the body is modified to accept the new information of the visions. But this is not always true. Sometimes baths are taken before the ceremony to open the person up, and sometimes they are taken by themselves, as a healing.

A tub is filled with water and to this is added the plants that the patient most needs, like mucura and ajo sacha, some of the most powerful doctors... The patient must approach in a sacred manner, in prayer that his needs will be met, and with the intention that they will. The shaman then pours the water over his head and lets it run down his body, also blowing him with smoke to purify him, or with perfume so he will flourish. Sometimes the patient turns as this is happening – first to the left [in a circle, anti-clockwise], then to the right [clockwise]. The first turn is to get rid of negativity; the second to draw in positivity. The bath takes place on the bank of a river so the energy that is removed will find its way to the sea [i.e. be taken away completely].

Floral baths do not usually contain large numbers of plants; rather, specific plants or flowers are chosen according to the patient's needs. The shaman begins by collecting fresh plants from the forest, then mashes up flowers and adds their juice to the mixture. During the entire process of collection, preparation and administering of baths to patients he must also follow the shamanic diet so that he, too, is pure. Artiduro continues:

> You can either have a one-off floral bath or a series of them for a deeper and more thorough effect. A common reason for people to want to take floral baths is that something is not going well for them – like, for example, they can't get work or they are having bad luck. First I give them a cleansing bath to take away the saladera [bad luck] which shows up as salt on their skins. In that bath I put ajo sacha, mishquipanga [*Renealmia alpine*], ruda [rue] and romero [rosemary]. Then [another bath, using different flowers and plants] follows to give the things the client wants: luck, work, etc.
>
> For changing luck, mucura is used and the patient will find that after a couple of weeks, things have changed. For example you may find the job you were looking for, or where your life felt stuck or turbulent there is some momentum; things start to shift. Mucura is also used for clearing negative thoughts and feelings sent to you by others. For cleansing the spirit, the dark red leaves of pinon colorado are used to undo sorcery and harm. This plant is also used in steam baths and when this is done you can actually see the phlegm, which is the bad magic, appear on the patient's skin as it comes out of the body. For flour-ishing or blossoming, *bano de florecimiento* plants are used.

These help us to connect with and draw upon the strength and courage within ourselves, to overcome obstacles, and to lead a purposeful and productive life in accordance with our soul's intention. The mixture for this bath is… water from a place in the forest where pure rainwater collects… To this is added albahaca [basil], which is a plant used widely in Peru for its strong, sweet perfume… From a floral bath perspective, it attracts lots of friends and positive outcomes. It is also used medicinally for gastritis, appendix, or gall bladder problems, in which case you can take it as a tea. Menta [mint] is also added to freshen and re-vitalise the bather. Menta is also good for calming the nerves and releasing worries and preoccupations. When the person bathes, all of these plant qualities are absorbed by the skin and the spirit.

Combination of Elements

In the next chapter we look at some of the healing successes of ayahuasca but, again, bear in mind that it is usually *all* of these elements – the bath, the diet, the energy of the shaman; indeed, even the effect of 'spiritual osmosis': taking in the power of the rainforest and the energies released during ceremony – which creates the healing. Although a powerful medicine in its own right, that is, it is not always ayahuasca that heals and it is rarely used by shamans alone. For the latter reason it may actually be difficult to assess what has caused the healing – ayahuasca or one of the other elements in the process? – but, still, there is no doubt that the vine of souls produces sometimes life-changing results.

2

Healing with Ayahuasca

I struggle to find words to describe the experience – it was beyond words: one of the most intense and exhilarating experiences I have had in my adult life. It allowed me to really connect at a deeper level whilst opening new doors, perceptions, realities, and opportunities I didn't consider possible. Would I do it again? Yes, next year! I'm already planning to return.
Alexia, United Kingdom[5]

The power of ayahuasca and the healing regime which surrounds it is encapsulated to some extent in the feedback I receive from participants on my retreats in Peru where we work with ayahuasceros in the Amazon and the San Pedro curanderos of the Andes. This is some of it:

This experience was one of the most transformative of my life and the healing and self-exploration I did was unlike any I have experienced before. It is impossible to describe what an ayahuasca journey is like but it is something that anyone on a voyage of self-discovery should consider. The jungle is awe-inspiring but it is in the journey that the true magic lies.
Eleanor Niblock, journalist, writing in *Green Events* magazine, UK

My last journey with the vine was so mind-blowingly beautiful that I laughed, danced and cried tears of sheer joy. It really let me see the beauty and magic of the world.
Ross, photographer, Scotland

The whole experience has profoundly enlightened and changed

me. I've just welled up with tears at the prospect of sharing it all again with you!
Emer, social worker, Ireland

I am the happiest man I know! I asked for love and received it! You can't imagine how Peru changed who I am and brought out the real me!
Heath, financial consultant, Australia

People ask 'How was the trip' – and what do you answer??? No words can do it justice. There are too many experiences – and none would shed light on my true feelings! The stillness I feel now and the lack of rush is incredible. What we experienced was something so special – and life just keeps getting better.
Linzi, health and fashion consultant and TV presenter, UK

An experience that changed my life for the better. It is hard to describe something so magical but I will draw from it for the rest of my days.
Annette, stables owner, USA

Ecstasy and euphoria rolled into one. Thank you from every depth of my heart for the loving, profound, and lasting healing I received. You gave me back my life.
Stafford, retired, UK

Ayahuasca was the most powerful medicine and marked the beginning of a new era of integrity for me. My whole life has shifted in fantastically powerful ways.
Marc, restaurant worker, Australia

In this chapter we look at healing with ayahuasca and I'll present a few deeper case studies to show how plants work their magic when Western medicines often fail.

My own introduction to ayahuasca was in 1998. Like many other dissatisfied Westerners, disillusioned with my job, my relationships, and feeling let down by the world in general, I made the pilgrimage to Peru to find new meaning and direction for my life. The story of my own adventure is told in my book *Drinking the Four Winds* so it's enough here to simply say that it worked, leading to a radical change in career and to a number of other decisions which shaped my life (and continue to) in a whole new way. What is more interesting here though is that on that first journey there was also a young woman at our retreat centre who had come for help with a serious physical problem. This was years ago and, sadly, I can't remember her name now so let's call her Gail.

Gail's Story

Gail was incredibly brave. She arrived in the jungle in a wheel-chair, a result of paralysis due to a brain tumour. She had undergone treatment for it, which had led to her hair falling out and problems with her skin, but it had not helped her at all. Eventually the treatment was discontinued and her doctors told her she now had just a few months to live.

This, incidentally, is a curse; something that Western doctors do often with their diagnoses and prognoses. We understand enough now about human psychology and 'obedience to authority' through the work of Milgram, Zimbardo and many more recent studies to know that the words of an 'expert' are often regarded not just as advice or information but as instructions and orders. Where people believe and accept them, as they usually do from an expert, the words themselves can create the very outcome they describe: a self-fulfilling prophecy. There are even cases of perfectly healthy people becoming seriously ill or worse because their doctor effectively told them to.[6] Just because an expert tells us something, however, it does not mean that it *has* to happen (as Gail's story suggests.) Nevertheless, she had come to the rainforest not so much expecting a cure but for an adventure in the final days of her life.

The shaman for our first ceremony was an ayahuascero called Javier. He was only contracted for one ceremony and then had to leave for appointments elsewhere while a new curandero joined our group. Something happened to Javier during that first ceremony though: having drunk ayahuasca he was visited by his spirits who told him that Gina could be cured and that he could cure her. So in the morning he cancelled his other engagements and asked if he could stay on with us. He didn't ask for further payments (although we paid him, of course), he just wanted to help. From that moment he became Gail's private physician while other shamans took over the ceremonies for the rest of our group as planned.

Javier worked tirelessly for Gail. Walking out into the jungle each morning to fetch fresh herbs for her treatments, he made a balm for her skin, a lotion for her scalp, and found medicines for her diet. In the evenings, following the guidance of his spirits, he held private ceremonies for her, delivering whatever healing was required.

We didn't see Gail all week but at the end of this period she re-emerged, and she was walking. She used a stick to steady herself and her movements were stiff but she was out of her wheelchair. Her skin was also noticeably improved, with no more dry patches and redness, and her hair was growing back, after one week to a length of an inch or so in contrast to almost total baldness before. When she returned home from Peru she went for a medical check-up and an X-ray confirmed that her tumour had shrunk in size.

This was an amazing success for Gail, for her healer and for ayahuasca, but before we get too carried away and start talking about 'miracle cures' I want to be clear that Gail still eventually died. It is important to keep a sense of perspective with ayahuasca healing, as I said at the beginning of this book.

What *is* significant, however, is that she lived for a further six years when her Western doctors had given her just a few weeks. She was able to enjoy those years too, as an independent woman, able to walk and care for herself, and with her beauty and freshness restored. She used her new lease of life to travel the world and have adventures and love affairs as any young woman might. When she died, she died happy; something her doctors would have denied her.

Tracie's Story

Tracie is an Australian woman with another success story to tell as a result of her recovery, through ayahuasca and other plants, from a quite different disease: alcoholism and drug addiction. She writes:[7]

I had a traumatic childhood which led to a 30-year relationship with drugs and alcohol.

I have used just about everything but my substance of choice was heroin. I used it on and off from the age of 16 until my last dabble at the age of 35. Every time I gave up heroin I did so using alcohol and I continued to be an addict for another 10 years...

It took me years to realise that I even had a problem and more years before I could feel my own emptiness. Then it dawned on me that I had nothing going on inside. Somewhere in the trauma of my childhood I had chosen not to feel and in that choosing I had lost touch with myself. I mistook the highs and lows of addiction, the flush of infatuation, the pride of the pay-packet and the thrill of anything fast or dangerous as true feeling and emotion... I was what therapists call a high-functioning addict. I've also had two successful seven-year relationships. One ended because of my heroin use and the last because of alcohol. I did a lot of running away...

I stayed in Korea for three years and in that time I was hospitalised twice, drunk and delusional, and was put into a mental

*institution where no-one spoke English. It was terrifying. Some
of the women there had been totally abandoned by their families
and left alone for 15 or 20 years. This was probably my lowest
point but I still had a few years of drinking to do before seeking
help. I was scared of myself and for myself...*

*Then one day I woke up and actually woke up. I realised that
this was it, my life, forever. I went straight to my doctor and
asked for help... the longest, hardest, most successful rehabilitation programme available. He told me that the success rate was
the same for all of them... 30 per cent.*

Shocked and dismayed at this low success rate she nonetheless
signed up for the toughest programme she could find: the 10-
month Bridge Program run by the Salvation Army. As it was to
turn out, Tracie was one of the lucky ones: the 30 per cent that
rehabilitation like this can help. The other nine women who
started the treatment with her were not so fortunate. 'After one
month we were down to seven; after three months we were
down to five and by the end of the sixth month there were just
three of us... Rachael, Kim and I were the lucky ones... we were
going to live free...'

Within two months of completing the programme however,
Rachael was dead. 'Cause: alcohol. She was a beautiful, lively,
funny 35-year-old and one of my main inspirations now for
seeking an alternative treatment for addiction. Kim is thankfully
still alive but hospitalised for alcohol-related issues. She tells me
she has good days and bad. So much for the magic 30 per cent.'
In Tracie's experience with Western treatments, then, 30 per cent
(which is low enough) is actually the best possible positive
outcome. In her group, at least, the real figure was 10 per cent.
Only she made it.

In Tracie's experience with Western treatments, then, 30 per
cent (which is low enough) is actually the *best* possible positive
outcome. In her group, at least, the real figure was 10 per cent.

Only she made it.

'There had to be a better way', she reasoned and, inspired to find it, she trained as a drug and alcohol counsellor and for the next two years threw herself into researching rehabilitation programmes worldwide, 'but no matter where I looked I could not find anything better than the 30 per cent success rate for addictions that I already knew and had experienced using standard Western methods.'

Then she came across an article about the Takiwasi Centre, in Peru, an addictions healing Centre claiming a 75 per cent success rate. That caught her attention but the only significant difference she could find between their approach and the Western model was the use of plant medicines. They used tobacco as a purgative and a plant she had never heard of – ayahuasca. She began looking for a way to get to Peru to experience the plant first-hand and eventually came across my website with details of the trips I run to the Amazon to work with the shamans there. She writes:

My introduction to plant medicines could not have been better. We did seven ayahuasca ceremonies in Iquitos and then travelled to Cusco for two ceremonies with wachuma, better known as San Pedro. I could see immediately what was missing in the Western rehabilitation model: the connection to spirit which both plants gave. Ayahuasca helped me find myself; San Pedro completed the process by reconnecting me with the world... This feeling of connectedness is something alien to addicts who often share a common grievance that they feel 'different' to their peers, their family and indeed to society as a whole. Now... I realised that we are all the same: energetic, spiritual beings; that our very breath intermingles with those around us as does the energy of our thoughts and words.

After the course ended Tracie returned briefly to Australia, but only to put her affairs in order, then she moved permanently to

Peru.

While I lived in Cusco I travelled regularly to the north of Peru for ceremonies and dietas with other plants too, including ayahuasca, guayusa, ajo sacha and bobinsena.[8] I met a number of shamans who were having success in treating addictions with plant medicines. The whole process was incredibly exciting to me. It was no longer just an idea that freedom from addiction was possible; it was actually happening for real people in Peru as a result of the plant medicines and shamanic practices there. I was amazed, awed and ecstatic. After years of searching I had found what I had been seeking.

In Pucallpa I met the shaman Jose Campos who had been one of the original founders of the Takiwasi Centre. He agreed to help me in any way he could and offered me sound advice about the use of plants for healing. In the village of San Francisco, just outside Pucallpa, I met another shaman, Mateo Arevalo, who is treating addicts in his home and having great success... Everywhere in Peru it seemed – from the mountains to the jungle – so many different shamans were having extraordinary success in healing addictions by using plant medicines. These were not 'freak incidents' or isolated cases of breakthroughs by addicts. The results were consistent and far superior to Western achievements...

After that life moved quickly. I wrote up an addictions treatment programme using plants, therapeutic practices and shamanic medicines which I called Tranquilo (Spanish for calm, peaceful and quiet), found a place to rent just outside Iquitos and had my first client booked before I'd even moved in.

Tracie's month-long *Tranquilo* programme includes an ayahuasca ceremony in week one, along with purges (plants that cause vomiting or other forms of release to remove toxins from the body), detoxifying saunas and plant baths. In week two there are daily meditation and counselling sessions and two more ayahuasca ceremonies. This continues in week three, with three more ayahuasca ceremonies. Then in week four San Pedro (a plant that connects us to the Earth, to ourselves and to love) is added to the programme and there are three ceremonies with it. As I said in the last chapter, healing with ayahuasca is typically (and more effectively) a *process* and not just a one-off ceremony.

The real purpose of Tranquilo is to find out who you truly are and all of the power, dignity and beauty you have. The Western social system that I was born into and lived within drilled into me that I was powerless and weak and taught me that evil exists and that society is fragmented – but none of that is actually true. We are powerful, beautiful and extraordinary. I know this through my work with plant teachers. There is no reason why we cannot find out for ourselves who we are and where we are going and no reason why any individual cannot be fully empowered and healed...

We weren't born as addicts, we were born as human beings and the whole process of becoming an addict is learned. Its purpose is to cover our sense of separation and the hurts we feel have been done to us in this game of life... If we only realised the truth of our relationship to each other, however, to nature and the extent of our power, then the entire manufactured structure of the society which causes these wounds would collapse like a house of cards. A new consciousness is already emerging that sees the world as a single organism and reason will tell you that an organism bent on damaging itself is doomed. Plants open doorways to this new consciousness and give us back our connection to the world...

I've been advised by the shamans I have met who treat addiction that it is not wise to consider plants as a miracle cure. I have also met addicts who have come to the Amazon with a miracle cure in mind only to find that they leave the jungle and the first thing they crave is a beer. In some cases one or two ceremonies may do the trick but don't bet on it. In my experience and in the experience of others, it takes time to assimilate the message of the plants. I believe ayahuasca can give us a deeply spiritual experience but this needs to be integrated and understood to have a lasting effect.

Kira's Story

Kira was not a student or a client of mine but a journalist for National Geographic magazine who visited Peru to look for a cure for her life-long depression. Her story (dramatically, but quite relevantly under the circumstances) is entitled *Hell and Back* and can be read in full at http://www.nationalgeographic.com /adventure/0603/features/peru.html. It is an interesting one because it illustrates much of what we have been talking about so far: the *process* of healing with ayahuasca and the elements that go into it. Of these, ayahuasca per se may not even be the most important although it is of course the core of the experience: the thing that holds everything else together and the reason why the healing will work at all.

Kira describes her problem, and the ayahuasca ceremony that finally cured it, as follows.

I will never forget what it was like. The overwhelming misery. The certainty of never-ending suffering. No one to help you, no way to escape. Everywhere I looked: darkness so thick that the idea of light seemed inconceivable. Suddenly, I swirled down a tunnel of fire, wailing figures calling out to me in agony, begging me to save them. Others tried to terrorize me. 'You will never leave here' they said. 'Never. Never'... the darkness became even thicker; the emotional charge of suffering nearly unbearable. I felt as if I would burst from heartbreak – everywhere, I felt the agony of humankind, its tragedies, its hatreds, its sorrows. I reached the bottom of the tunnel and saw three thrones in a black chamber. Three shadowy figures sat in the chairs; in the middle was what I took to be the devil himself. 'The darkness will never end,' he said. 'It will never end. You can never escape this place.'

'I can,' I replied. All at once, I willed myself to rise. I sailed up through the tunnel of fire, higher and higher until I broke through to a white light. All darkness immediately vanished. My body felt light, at peace. I floated among a beautiful spread of colours and patterns. Slowly my ayahuasca vision faded. I returned to my body, to where I lay in the hut... The next morning, I discovered the impossible: The severe depression that had ruled my life since childhood had miraculously vanished... With shamanism − and with the drinking of ayahuasca in particular − I've learned that, for me, the worse the experience, the better the payoff. There is only one requirement for this work: You must be brave. You'll be learning how to save yourself.

That, however, is the *end* of her story. Typically this drama, excitement and eventual triumph is all we get from many other accounts of healings with ayahuasca − which is why we must be careful about taking them only at face value, because, as Kira goes on to explain, what actually produced her healing was far more than a single cupful of ayahuasca.

Kira grew up among 'fundamentalist atheists', she says, who taught her that 'we're all alone in the universe, the fleeting dramas of our lives culminating in a final, ignoble end: death. Nothing beyond that.' As she concludes: 'It was not a prescription for happiness.'

I'll say. And yet this fascination for (or habit of) separation is so prevalent as to be the norm in the Western world. Human beings have become habituated (or, more cynically, indoctrinated) to see themselves as, among other things, separate from God (our religious 'industry' demands it so that our priests − God's CEOs − can offer us salvation at a price), separate from nature (any number of businesses benefit from this illusion – or delusion: from oil companies, GM food producers and pharmaceutical firms who exploit the planet because of it, to Greenpeace and Friends of the Earth at the other end of the scale who exist to protect us from the former, and somewhere in the middle are businesses like urban zoos and factory farms which present us with animals for our entertainment or consumption). As our communities have broken down we are now even separate from each other.

This, however, is rarely seen as a (wholly) bad thing. The very idea of separation is, after all, bound up in our myths of glory, in the form of the 'lone hero', the 'masked man', the 'outsider', the 'rebel' or the 'saviour'. All of them stand alone and save the day. The real and non-heroic consequence of this, however, is the point that Tracie makes, above: for her it led to years of misery as a drunk and a drug addict; in my experience, it is one of the primary causes of all of our Western soul sicknesses.

Disease, as any shaman will tell you – even if it eventually manifests as a brain tumour, addiction, an ulcer, diabetes, or another physical problem – arises from a soul that is in some way imbalanced. By separating ourselves from the source of our power (whether we see that power as 'God' or 'purpose', 'love' or 'passion' or some other positive force) weakens us and makes our soul an easy target for another 'spirit' to attack. A Western doctor might call it 'depression', 'chronic fatigue syndrome' or some other label instead of a 'spirit', but the point is really the same. Unless we remove the negative force that grips us, and recharge ourselves from a source of power, our problems really begin.

Kira's problem was that the world seemed:

...a dark, forbidding place beyond my control. And my mortality gaped at me mercilessly.

... there were [also] some stubborn enemies hiding out in my

psyche: Fear and Shame... How do you describe what it's like to want love from another but to be terrified of it at the same time? To want good things to happen to you, while some disjointed part of you believes that you don't deserve them? To look in a mirror and see only imperfections? This was the meat and potatoes of my several years of therapy. Expensive therapy. Who did what, when, why. The constant excavations of memory. The sleuth-work. Patching together theory after theory. Rational-emotive behavioural therapy. Gestalt therapy. Humanistic therapy. Biofeedback. Positive affirmations: I am a beautiful person. I deserve the best in life. Then, there's the impatience. Thirty-three years old already, for chrissakes' – and nothing so far had cured her depression.

Kira describes one of her early ayahuasca ceremonies as follows:

Soon I start to see a pale green glow; colourful, primordial forms, resembling amoebas or bacteria, float by. Alarmed, I open my eyes. And this is uncanny: I can see the rafters of the hut, the thatch roof, the glow of the stars outside the screened windows – but the same amoeba-like things are passing over that view, as if superimposed. 'You're seeing with your third eye,' one of the apprentices explains... Fantastical scenes glide by, composed of ever-shifting geometric forms and textures. Colours seem to be the nature of these views; a dazzling and dizzying display of every conceivable hue blending and parting in kaleidoscopic brilliance.

But then the colours vanish all at once as if a curtain has been pulled down. Blackness. Everywhere. Dark creatures sail by. Tangles of long, hissing serpents. Dragons spitting fire. Screaming humanlike forms. For a bunch of hallucinations, they seem terrifyingly real. An average ayahuasca ceremony lasts about four to five hours. But in ayahuasca space – where time, linear thought, and the rules of three-dimensional reality no longer apply – four to five hours of sheer darkness and terror can feel like a lifetime. My heartbeat soars; it's hard to breathe... what I'm experiencing now is my fear taking symbolic form through the ayahuasca. Fear that I have lived with my entire life and that needs to be released... I work on controlling my breathing. But such thick darkness. Clouds of bats and demonlike faces. Black lightning. Black walls materializing before me no matter which way I turn. Closer and closer, the darkness surrounding me, trapping me. I can barely breathe.

At this point Kira called out for help from her shaman, Hamilton. His response is typical of the shamanic approach to healing in ceremony and illustrates once again that it is not just ayahuasca which produces a cure, but a number of interconnected actions and energies, including the visions themselves and what they reveal, the intent of the shaman to heal and the patient to be healed, the energies contained in the songs of the shaman, and the other plant allies which he may call into the ceremony.

Hamilton is standing over me now, rattling his chacapa, singing his spirit songs. Inexplicably, as he does this, the darkness backs off.[9] But more of it comes in a seemingly endless stream. I see dark, raging faces. My body begins to contort; it feels as if little balls are ripping through my flesh, bursting from my skin. The pain is excruciating. I writhe on the mattress, screaming. Hamilton calls over one of his helpers – a local woman named Rosa – with directions to hold me down.

And now [the spirits] appear to be escaping en masse from my throat. I hear myself making otherworldly squealing and hissing sounds. Such high-pitched screeches that surely no human could ever make. All the while there is me, like a kind of witness, watching and listening in horror, feeling utterly helpless to stop it. I've read nothing about this sort of experience happening when taking ayahuasca.

This is a good point. Many of the accounts of 'miracle cures' and 'life-changing encounters' with ayahuasca that I have also read tend to focus on the beauty of the imagery and ignore completely what it is to be *really* healed. Situations like the one that Kira experienced can and do happen though. Not always, but sometimes. (See my book *Drinking the Four Winds* for examples of the exorcisms and spirit battles I have been involved with in my ceremonies in Peru.)

> *On and on it goes. The screaming, the wailing. My body shakes wildly; I see a great serpent emerging from my body, with designs on Hamilton. He shakes his chacapa at it, singing loudly, and after what seems like an infinite battle of wills, the creature leaves me. I grab the vomit bucket and puke for several minutes. Though my stomach has been empty for over eight hours, a flood of solid particles comes out of me… The visions fade. My body stops shaking… The shamans believe that what we vomit out during a ceremony is the physical manifestation of dark energy and toxins being purged from the body. The more that comes out, the better.*

The process of healing continued for Kira (once again, one drink of ayahuasca seldom does the trick) and even:

> *After three ceremonies, I still feel that I have something big to purge… We begin the ceremony, drink the ayahuasca. I'm hoping to find myself in some heavenly realms this time, but again, as usual, the darkness. With disappointment, I find myself entering a familiar tunnel of fire, heading down to one of the hell realms. I don't know where I'm going, or why, when I suddenly glimpse the bottom of the tunnel and leap back in shock: Me, I'm there, but as a little girl. She's huddled, captive, in a ball of fire before the three thrones of the devil and his sidekicks. As soon as I reach her, she begins wailing, 'Don't leave me! Don't leave me!'*

I think this must be a part of me that I lost. Long ago. The shamans believe that whenever a traumatic event happens to us, we lose part of our spirit, that it flees the body to survive the experience. And that unless a person undergoes a shamanistic 'soul retrieval' these parts will be forever lost. Each one, they say, contains an element of who [we] truly are; people may lose their sense of humour, their trust of others, their innocence...
'The darkness was so heavy during your childhood,' a spirit voice says to me 'that your soul splintered beneath the weight.'

With encouragement from her shaman, Kira is able to reach down and take the hand of her child-self. 'When she feels my touch, she stops crying, and I pull her up, out of the tunnel of fire. The darkness departs. We reach realms of bright white light – the first such places my visions have allowed. The heavenly realms.'

In her final ceremony, despite her soul retrieval, 'Darkness falls' again.

A scathing pain rises in my chest – the most excruciating pain I've ever felt...

Legions of demons sail out of my body. I'm helpless before them; they contort me. I'm made to see that what is being purged now is a deeply rooted belief that I don't deserve to be alive, that no one can love me and I will always need to justify my existence. Slowly I gain the upper hand over the darkness and order it to leave my body. I feel a pressure in my chest that could break all my ribs. I grab my bucket, vomit out what appears to be a stream of fire. Hamilton kneels down and blows tobacco smoke onto the top of my head. I cough violently and watch as demons burst out of me, roaring, only to disintegrate in white light.

And [then] before me [is] this enormous image of God. He takes me in his arms and coddles me like a child. I know, unequivocally, that I am loved and have always been loved. That I matter and have always mattered. That I'm safe and, no matter what happens, will always be safe. I will never allow myself to become separated from him again.

Of course, a single drink of ayahuasca might solve all your problems – Pablo Amaringo, the visionary artist and one-time ayahuascero writes, for example,[10] that: 'I became a shaman when I saw a curandera heal my younger sister by using ayahuasca. My sister had been in agony with hepatitis but with this single healing from the plants she was cured in just two hours… Later I began dieting and taking la purga and she taught me how to use plants for healing' – but it didn't happen for any of the people mentioned in this chapter – for Gail, Tracie or Kira – and in my experience it's rare. Your *dedication to healing* – your *intention to be well* – and your willingness to do whatever it takes count for a lot; much more in fact than giving away your power (which also includes your *healing* power) to a shaman and a cup of jungle brew or a Western doctor and a 'magical pill' for that matter. But there are exceptions, as Pablo's story shows.

How Shamanic/Ayahuasca/Amazonian Healing Works

It should be clear by now that shamanic healing has a very different view of the nature and causes of illness than orthodox Western medicine. For one thing, the latter intervenes only at the point where the disease has become visible and rarely addresses the underlying cause, while shamanism aims to intervene at the point of the cause so the underlying issues are dealt with.

For the shaman, there are a number of ways in which disease might arise but in every case there is an unseen world where all illness comes from and from where it can migrate to the physical plane as a result of magical or spiritual actions or distress. In this system disease manifests along these lines:

(4) Physical (the seen world)
▲

(3) Mental
▲

(2) Emotional
▲

(1) Spiritual (the unseen world)

At the root of every illness is a problem that stems from spirit and affects our spiritual bodies first. In Kira's case, growing up with 'fundamentalist atheists' and their indoctrination that, 'We're all alone in the universe, the fleeting dramas of our lives culminating in a final, ignoble end: death. Nothing beyond that,' was enough to frighten and damage her. 'It was not a prescription for happiness.'

In Peru, there is a condition called *susto*: soul loss caused by fright, which particularly affects children since their souls are more fluid and less attached to the physical body than an adult's. An unkind or unthinking word, idea or action can therefore cause it to take flight to escape a condition that it finds terrifying or intolerable. Kira's parents may not have set out to frighten her (how many parents really *intend* to damage their kids?) but through their insistence on a Godless universe and a life of aloneness followed by death, that is what they did.

This 'soul sickness' then begins its migration from the 'immaterial world' to the physical body and is registered next by the emotions. If we are in tune with our feelings we may sense that there is something 'not quite right' with us at this stage, although we may still be unable to articulate what the problem is or how we are really feeling.

As the illness becomes more solid and physical, however, we also become increasingly aware that something is wrong. At this point the illness is entering the mental self and the mind goes to work on the problem so we become consciously aware of some event or trauma that haunts us and seems to have a connection to our feelings and illness, or perhaps our mind also becomes affected by the spiritual fallout from that event, in which case mental illness, anxiety, depression or some other illness might result. Finally, the spiritual issue will create a physical problem.

In my book *Medicine for the Soul* I give the example of stress as a modern form of soul sickness. In fact, there is no such thing as 'A Stress' (the term was only invented less than 100 years ago). You cannot examine it in the way you can a broken leg for example; it exists in the world of the unseen; it is a mood, a sense, a feeling – a spirit (of the workplace, a relationship or a life circumstance for example). Yet many of us are affected by stress emotionally and mentally, leading to relationship problems, anguish, anger, panic attacks and depression. Eventually, when our coping strategies run out and our emotional and mental selves cannot deal with it any longer, stress begins assaulting the physical body and is nowadays recognised even by orthodox medical professionals as a contributor to cancers, strokes, ulcers, heart attacks, hypertension and many other organic problems as well as numerous secondary ones, such as the impact on our health of increased smoking, drinking and eating disorders and decreased sex drive and life force. And yet stress does not exist in a literal way! It is the invisible world making itself felt on the visible.

Because all illness has a spiritual cause, in this way the shaman understands that its cure also lies in the spiritual domain. There may be many ways in which these spiritual problems arise, however, and to understand them and their cures the shaman must also know the workings of the soul since this is the part of us that suffers first.

The Soul

The scientific and medical community is sceptical about the idea of a soul since it cannot be seen, quantified, analysed or measured in the way of the physical sciences. But even a hardened sceptic might nowadays concede that most of what we think of as 'solid' (including ourselves) is actually *bits* of material held together by energetic forces – the discoveries of atomic and quantum physics have taught us that much. Perhaps only the terminology is different. The shaman calls this energy 'soul' but his approach is in many ways the same as the scientist; both are manipulating forces that cannot be seen to create material changes in the world which can.

Because he is an expert in the nature and workings of the soul the shaman is aware of its subtleties and flow. In fact he may even conceive of these subtleties as a number of different souls, not just one. The Shipibos of the Amazon for example believe that every part of the human body and every organ has its own soul.[11] It is all of these souls together that form *the soul*. Thus, for example, a physical accident such as a broken arm can lead to that soul part leaving the body in shock and, even when the arm is treated and healed, feeling may not return to it until its missing soul is recovered. And since the soul of that body part also contributes to the whole, the rest of us will be energetically depleted too while it remains missing.

When we lose some of our power in this way we are less able to defend ourselves against other spiritual forces and are open to attack from entities that are energetically out of resonance with us. In a case such as Kira's, where it was not her arm but her heart or her spirit that was broken, this power-loss might even lead to a possession state where, in psychological terms, part of our personality or self is no longer under our control but fulfilling its own agenda and driving us to act in a way which is not in our interests. In shamanic terms, this is the result of a spirit intrusion and it may require an exorcism to remove it, as was the case for Kira.

Spirit Intrusions

Spirit intrusions are really power intrusions. As the anthropologist Michael Harner puts it: 'They are not natural to the body, but are brought in. If you are power-full, you will resist them... Serious illness is usually only possible when a person is dis-spirited, has lost this energizing force, the guardian spirit. When a person becomes depressed, weak, prone to illness, it is a symptom that he has lost his power... and thus can no longer resist, or ward off the unwanted 'infections' or intrusions.'

In psychological terms, we might say, for example, that the 'fundamentalist' and forcefully held views of Kira's parents were a power that they held over her and a belief system that she became infected with. Since they were not her own views to begin with, and nor did they help her, she could not fully accept them, however, and the dissonance this caused led to a troubled mind and eventually to depression. The shamanic view is actually not that different.

In shamanic terms, the intrusion that invades you begins its life as a form of energy (or spirit) but soon develops an awareness of its own and a will to live, becoming more and more physical as it does so. (In other words, an *idea* gathers strength when we act on it in the world. It then becomes a *behaviour pattern* which, in turn, reinforces the belief: a vicious circle.) If its drive-to-life is stronger than your drive to resist it, it will eventually develop an independent material presence, fuelling itself by drawing from your energy so that to all intents and purposes it possesses you.

The notions that 'illness is usually only possible when a person is dis-spirited' and that, 'If you are power-full [i.e. filled with your own power and not the disabling power or ideas of somebody else], you will resist [such illness],' is not at all fantastical, by the way. Indeed, science offers some support for this view. In a number of experiments it has been shown, for example, that people who are weaker and less power-filled are also less resistant to disease. The psychologists Holmes and Rahe found that the most stressful life events – those which bring us down, depress us or leave us in a weakened state – such as bereavement, divorce, redundancy or retirement – *always* correlate with the onset of illness. In one experiment two groups of people – those under stress and those with a non-stressful life – were asked to inhale a cold virus. Those who were stressed caught colds within days while those who were happy with their lives did not get ill at all. Another experiment showed that people under stress always develop throat infections when a virus is circulating and consistently do so within four days of exposure to it.

What science is acknowledging in such studies is almost a latent endorsement of the shaman's view that being power-full will prevent disease and ward off spiritual attack while emotional and spiritual weakness gives the disease the foothold it needs.

When physical illness does result therefore it will rarely be the shaman's primary (or at least not his only) concern since he knows that by dealing with the point of origination and the cause of the disease (the intrusive spirit or disabling idea and the circumstances that admitted it) he will also heal its manifestations in the emotional, mental and physical bodies. The most important thing then, is to extract the harmful spirit (or damaging energy) from his client. When this is done the client's energy body will reconstitute itself to close the gap left by the intrusion and her own power will begin to circulate again.

Kira's shaman explained it to her in this way: 'Everyone has an energetic body run by an inextinguishable life force. In Eastern traditions, this force, known as chi or prana, is manipulated through such things as acupuncture or yoga to run smoothly and prevent the build-up of the negative energies that cause bodily disease, mental illness, and even death. To Amazonian shamans, however, these negative energies are actual spirit entities that attach themselves to the body and cause mischief. In everyone, there is a loving 'higher self' but whenever unpleasant thoughts enter a person's mind – anger, fear, sorrow – it's because a dark spirit is hooked to the body and is temporarily commandeering the person's mind.'

Spirit Extraction

The method of spirit extraction (or exorcism) is consistent across shamanic cultures. Usually it involves finding a replacement host for the spirit of the disease so it can be removed from the client's body. In *Drinking the Four Winds*, for example, I wrote about an exorcism I performed for a client during an ayahuasca ceremony.

Earlier that day myself and the resident shaman at my healing centre in Peru had met with a client of ours, Jimmy, who had joined us for help with addictions, phobia and social anxiety, and during our discussions I had seen something on him – some energy which to me looked like a huge black tic attached to his belly[12]: some negative thoughtform that was sucking energy parasitically from him and which needed to be removed. The shaman couldn't see it. 'I only see spirits when I have drunk Ayahuasca,' he remarked, so I had asked him to look for it in the ceremony that night, which he did. At some point in the ceremony, however, all Hell broke loose.

I had noticed the presence of some pretty ugly energies in our moloka[13] during the healing for Jimmy, but I thought they were contained. Our shaman had been working on him as we'd agreed and had been removing all sorts of unwholesome energies in the form of snakes, beetles, scorpions and other unpleasant-looking entities which were now coursing around us. For my part I had been gathering them up as he pulled them out, wrestling them back into pure energy and throwing them out into the jungle where they could be re-absorbed by the Earth.

It dawned on me now however that there were an awful lot of them and maybe they weren't as contained as I'd thought. Just as that idea occurred to me I heard our shaman calling and his voice sounded weak. 'I saw that thing on Jimmy that you pointed out today and I removed it,' he said, after I had crawled my way to him. 'But there was a lot more beneath it which it was holding in,' he added. It appeared that he had – literally – opened a can of worms. 'And now there is this...' he said, pointing to Jimmy.

What I saw was a large dark form standing over our client. It looked reptilian and insect-like all at once and it was growling, snarling and angry. The shaman had been fighting it for hours and it had been spitting some form of 'evil' at him, as he called it; like smaller flying beetles, making them enter his throat so they could eat his songs, blocking his icaros to make him powerless against it. He needed to recover his strength so while he rested I took over the fight.

A spirit language began to work through me, becoming a song, a direction of energy that took on its own form and shape, like chains wrapping themselves around the entity Jimmy carried... a force to be spat out as an energy dart into the body of the creature before me; a poison arrow, carried on the breath. I kept up the song, accompanied by chacapa blows, for what seemed like an age before Jimmy began to vomit. The purge is a release of negativity. In the spirit world I was killing the demon inside him. In the physical world Jimmy was letting go of his sickness.

The entity looked weaker and then, out of nowhere, a voice spoke to me. 'Use tobacco,' it said. 'Blow smoke into it.' Just as I thought that, an assistant who had been sitting next to Jimmy throughout lit a mapacho and handed it to me. I blew the smoke into him where it formed a bubble, a cage, around the spirit inside him and then began to contract, tightening its grip. His demon was choking to death. And then a song, fully formed – the icaro de tobacco – began to sing itself through me: a warning to the invading spirit that, 'The smoke has you now and you will die unless you leave this body. What do you want to do?'

It nodded, weak, unable even to speak, but indicating its

willingness to go. At this point I thrust my hands into Jimmy's belly and gathered it up, throwing it out into the jungle where the energy that it represented landed in a tree. That tree, just outside the moloka, previously strong and healthy, was dead by morning.

In this case the tree became the new host for the entity or energy that Jimmy was carrying so he didn't have to, but other shamans use other objects or forms. Some Amazonian shamans told Peter Gorman, for example, author of *Ayahuasca in My Blood*, that they use a 'red room' – a spirit-space in another dimension – as a home for these beings and this is where they place them when they remove them from a client during a healing.

Restoring Power

Understandably, since the intrusion has been feeding off that person's energy or soul, part of her power will have been taken from her and it may be necessary to carry out a further healing to undo the damage caused by the intrusive spirit and fill the void in her energy body caused by the extraction.

'Core shamans'[14] call this 'power retrieval' and have a process for it which typically involves 'journeying' to the 'lower world' to find an 'animal spirit' as a source of power for the client. This may be helpful as a sort of psychological boost to that client, but it is not a form of healing known in the Amazon.

In Peru, the icaro is more likely to do the work of re-empowering the client, including special chants called *arkanas* which fill the person with power and form a magical shield of protection around them, or ayahuasca itself may empower the client during successive journeys from darkness to light, as was the case for Kira. Another option would be to put the client on a plant diet so that she could receive the specific power she needs in the form of a new ally: chuchuhuasi for love and connection, for example, or mucura as a further defence against power intrusions, sorcery and negative energy.

The Western Perspective on Ayahuasca Healing

As part of her National Geographic article, Kira reports how, in 1993, Charles Grob, MD launched the Hoasca Project, the first in-depth study of the physical and psychological effects of ayahuasca on humans. Grob's team studied members of the União do Vegetal (UDV) church in Brazil (a sort of fusion, like Santo Daime, of jungle medicine and Christianity), who use ayahuasca as a sacrament, comparing them to a control group that had never drunk ayahuasca.

The results showed that UDV members experienced recovery from addictions, depression and anxiety disorders more frequently and with more lasting effects than the normal population (control group). Their blood samples also showed that ayahuasca gives users a greater sensitivity to serotonin (a mood-regulating chemical produced by the body) by increasing the number of serotonin receptors on nerve cells.

'Ayahuasca is perhaps a far more sophisticated and effective way to treat depression than SSRIs [antidepressant drugs],' said Grob. 'It also has potential as a long-term solution.' SSRIs tend to suppress or mask the problem itself so we do not feel so depressed, but at the cost of making us less able to feel anything. Then, when the treatment is stopped, the old feelings return with full force. Doctors have also noticed with SSRIs that there is a window of some weeks after the patient first starts taking them when suicide due to depression is actually *more* likely since feelings of despair do not vanish immediately; the patient, however, now has more energy to act upon them. Thankfully, the same cannot be said for ayahuasca.

As well as these biochemical effects, the visions we receive from ayahuasca – and the process by which we come to them – are healing in themselves, in a way that Western medications are not. Grob sees this process – the state of profoundly altered consciousness in which visions occur – as a form of temporary 'ego disintegration' which allows people to move beyond their defence mechanisms and into their unconscious minds, showing them their deep thoughts and conditioning – the belief systems and self-limitations which can lead to illness. This, he says, is a unique opportunity which cannot be got at all from Western drugs or therapeutic methods. '[When] you come back with images, messages, even communications,' he says, 'You're learning about yourself, reconceptualising prior experiences. Having had a profound psycho-spiritual epiphany, you're not the same person you were before.'

He adds, however, that 'Ayahuasca is not for everyone... You have to be willing to have a very powerful, long, internal experience, which can get very scary. You have to be willing to withstand that.' The thing is though that by being willing to do so you may actually *heal* instead of perpetuating your sickness by masking it with SSRIs and other drugs which make you less present in the world and actually, therefore, less *alive*.

Dr Benny Shanon of the Hebrew University in Jerusalem has a rather different view, however. Shanon drank ayahuasca in more than 130 ceremonies and has also studied the accounts of others (several thousand in all) to produce his highly detailed book, *The Antipodes of the Mind*. His conclusion is that ayahuasca visions are not healing experiences so much as 'hallucinations', although he concedes that they are 'of the highest order'.

'I do not believe that there are beings and creatures just like us who reside elsewhere in other realms,' he says. Instead, 'Under [ayahuasca] intoxication, people's imagination and creative powers are greatly enhanced. Thus, their minds are prone to create the fantastic images they see.'

Even if Shanon is right, however (though I doubt it), it is my view that, for a (Western) culture unused to using our creative minds and more dependent each day on rational, analytical thinking, even an expansion in consciousness via an 'hallucination' can have a therapeutic effect. In her books, *Life Choices, Life Changes* and *The Joy of Burnout*, for example, Dr Dina Glouberman writes about what she calls 'Imagework': the utilisation of healing images coaxed from the unconscious (in her case, without the use of ayahuasca) which in themselves have led to profound break-throughs for people suffering the effects of trauma, abuse and even physical problems like cancer. In the second of her books she discusses how Imagework saved her life, in fact, by alerting her to her imminent death as a result of stress-related burnout. In this sense, even if ayahuasca 'only' provides us with greater access to our own unconscious (and not to spirit worlds), the healing it gives us can still save our lives (and our souls).[15]

Shanon may also be unique in his views about the more limited effects of the brew since, as Kira points out, 'Most ayahuasca researchers agree that, curiously, the compound appears to affect people on three different levels – the physical, psychological, and spiritual.' Although this may complicate the researchers' efforts to 'definitively catalog its effects, let alone explain specific therapeutic benefits', the point is that it *works* – and more deeply on us than just the mind. As Ralph Metzner, psychologist, ayahuasca researcher, and editor of the book *Sacred Vine of Spirits*, pointed out to Kira: '[Healing with ayahuasca] presumes a completely different understanding of illness and medicine than we are accustomed to in the West. But even from the point of view of Western medicine and psychotherapy it is clear that remarkable physical healings and resolutions of psychological difficulties can occur with this medicine.'

Dr Dennis McKenna (brother of Terence) has a more philo-sophical perspective on ayahuasca, having drunk it many times and also written about it from a purely scientific view. His conclusion, in his book, *The Brotherhood of the Screaming Abyss*, is much like my own: that it's not an either/or situation where we can believe in spirit worlds *or* the power of the mind to create states of healing. There is no contradiction at all in believing in both.

Of these spirit worlds he writes that, 'The ayahuasca

landscape is a virtual battleground populated with malevolent spirits but also with allies, plant teachers, animal spirits, guides, ancestral spirits and other morally ambiguous entities. The shaman's task is essentially one of extra-dimensional diplomacy, that is, to identify and form alliances with the beneficial entities while guarding against those that don't necessarily have one's best interests in mind.'

On the other hand, even in everyday life, 'Consciousness or mind forms the primary ground of being, while the physical world is secondary – a construct created by the mind. Any Eastern spiritual tradition or philosophy will tell you this is the case. Western thought, with its emphasis on materialism, is uncomfortable with that notion. I'm not aware of any finding in current neuroscience that resolves this question, at least not yet; but we do know enough about brain function to say with fair confidence that, to some extent, the world we call 'reality' is a construct of our brains. The brain assembles a coherent story (more or less)[16] by combining sensory experience with memories, associations, interpretations and intuitions, then presenting the result as the movie, or perhaps more accurately, the hallucination we inhabit [i.e. the trance state of everyday life]. If psychedelics teach us anything it's how fragile this constructed reality is.'

He summarises the two positions (mind or spirit) in the following way:

Possibility number one is that there actually are other dimensions, parallel realities that these substances [ayahuasca and other psychedelics] render accessible by temporarily altering our neurochemistry and perceptual apparatus. According to this model, there really are entities that want to communicate with us, or at least don't spurn communication when we poke our heads into their dimension. This is very close to the understanding of reality that prevails in most shamanic worldviews.

Possibility number two is the more parsimonious explanation, but it is almost as bizarre: For some reason, our brains have evolved the innate capability to generate three-dimensional visions of indescribable complexity and beauty, and that in... tryptamine states are presented to our inner perception accompanied by a sense of great emotional and intellectual import, and often seem to be narrated by a helpful entity, or entities that are perceived as distinct from the self.

Whether the first or second postulate is true, the conclusions from either are rather earth-shattering. If the first is true, then we are forced to reject, or at least radically revise, everything we think we know about reality. It makes our current models hopelessly obsolete and incomplete. All of human knowledge, all of our science and religion must be re-examined in the light of the understanding that our cosmic neighbourhood just 'over there' is of a completely different ontological order and, moreover, an order that is inhabited by entities as intelligent as we are, or many times more intelligent, but that share with us the quality of consciousness, of mindedness. And they are entities that want to share their reality with us, their wisdom, their knowledge, perhaps even form a symbiotic partnership or some form of diplomatic relationship. Whatever 'they' are, they do not seem to be hostile, and they appear to take a compassionate interest in our species, much as an adult might want to love and nurture a child.

On the other hand, if the second case is true, then the question stares us in the face: Why? Why in the course of neural evolutionary history has the brain developed the neural architecture and systems to sustain such experiences?' Perhaps so that this latent ability, activated through the ingestion of psychedelic substances, would give us the capability to manipulate images and symbols, he suggests. Through this, language could develop so that the symbols we work with can become even more complex and transglobal, leading eventually to our ability to move beyond the planet altogether and into the universe itself. 'If humanity is to have a destiny beyond the current dreary prospect of proliferating population and increasingly rapid strangulation of our planetary life support systems, this must surely be it.'

As I have written elsewhere (also see the next chapter), the spiritual purpose of ayahuasca is evolutionary: to take us out of ourselves and our limited beliefs of illness, separation and meaningless existence, into a universe filled with potential, and not just in an 'inner' personal healing sense, but *actually to the stars*. 'This passage is literally the birth canal leading to a new age, beyond history, beyond death, beyond time,' says McKenna.

Conclusion

In conclusion, then, you can believe what you like about ayahuasca: that it takes us to healing dimensions where plant doctors and spirit surgeons are waiting to work on us and heal our problems, or that it takes us deeper into ourselves where our own unconscious and remarkable innate powers of healing perform this magic instead.

In my view there is no contradiction between them. Ayahuasca does both – and more. But the bigger and more important point is this (to paraphrase one of my teachers): that if you desperately needed healing and ayahuasca provided it, you probably wouldn't bother to question why or how. The fact that it worked at all would be enough.

But all of this is just words on a page; there is no book on Earth that can give you the *experience* of ayahuasca. You simply have to join the ceremony and drink it. Then you find out for yourself.

3

Ayahuasca Origins and Visions

I was in absolute awe of the abilities of the shamans, who seemed able to look into my soul like an X-ray and use their icaros to knit back together the frayed edges. It seemed as though they were using an incredibly advanced technology not of this planet.
AJ, United Kingdom[17]

Where does ayahuasca come from? What are its origins and what is its purpose on Earth? Nobody really knows the answer to the first question but there are plenty of myths about the vine – ancient as well as modern – which provide us with a context to its use and which may help us answer our other questions.

In scientific terms, the vine itself is an inhibitor which contains harmala and harmaline, while chacruna contains vision-inducing alkaloids. It is the mixture of these that gives ayahuasca its unique properties. To put this another way, and to clear up one of the confusions which some people have about ayahuasca, it is not the vine which provides the visionary effects, but the plant, chacruna, which contains the visionary component: dimethyltryptamine (DMT).

If chacruna was taken by itself, however, pretty much nothing would happen because an enzyme in our stomachs, monoamine oxidase, would render its DMT content inert. The vine, however, contains monoamine oxidase inhibitors (MAOIs) in the form of harmine compounds, so when the two plants come together they complement each other and a psychoactive compound results, which also has an identical chemical make-up to the organic tryptamines in our bodies. The mixture is therefore able to make its way easily into our brains and bonds smoothly to our synaptic receptor sites, allowing a slow release of tryptamines into our bodies and a powerful visionary experience.

This is quite sophisticated chemistry given that it was discovered by rainforest tribes some 4,000 years ago or more, especially as modern science only began to understand the process itself in the 1950s. Which begs the question: How did the shamans know what they were doing and which plants to combine?

The answer provided by scientists is normally something along the lines of 'trial and error', but I have two problems with this: (1) There are some 150,000 species of plants in our rainforests and to try them all in combination to gain a visionary outcome would have taken years. I am not a mathematician but the possible combinations must surely run into millions. Furthermore, the vine and the chacruna plant do not grow anywhere near each other or look anything alike, so the shaman would have had no obvious indicator that the two would work together in the way that they do. (2) Moreover, however, the scientific answer is tautological in that it assumes that these combinations were tried and tested to arrive at a known effect – but how *could* this effect be known or sought after unless it *already* existed so the shamans knew what they were trying to replicate?

Asking the shamans themselves how they knew which plants to use often gets you the answer, 'Simple. The spirits told us,' which may appear to advance our understanding no further – unless, of course, you are prepared to take the shamans at their word, in which case this Shipibo legend may explain how ayahuasca came to be.[18]

There was once a woman who was interested in plants and liked to pick their leaves. She would crush them in a pot and soak them in water overnight. Then she would bathe in them each morning[19] before sunrise, knowing that the way to find out about plants and their effects is to be with them. One night she had a dream where an old woman came to her and asked, 'Why are you bathing in these leaves each day?'

The younger woman recognized her visitor as the spirit of the leaves. 'I am doing this because I want you to teach me', she answered. The older woman said, 'Then you must seek out my uncle. His name is Kamarampi. I will show you where to find him'.[20]

The young woman went to the uncle and he showed her how to pick the leaves of chacruna, which was the bush she had taken leaves from to bathe in. He showed her where to find ayahuasca, which is the lover of chacruna, and how to prepare a marriage of them both. He told her to tell the people how to celebrate this marriage and how to use the brew.

In other words, it was a dream – a message from the spirit world or the unconscious – which led to the discovery of ayahuasca. Such forms of communication, as surprising as it may seem, have been used by scientists as well and have led to some of our greatest breakthroughs. It was a dream state (aided by LSD) which enabled Crick and Watson to finally understand the structure of DNA, and a series of visions which also led the Nobel Prize winner Kary Mullis to come up with PCR, a technique for measuring 'viral load' which is used in the treatment of HIV and AIDS.

Another Amazonian legend, related by Javier, is that the first shamans drank their ayahuasca without chacruna until the vine showed them that its lover, the leaves, was missing. 'The ayahuasca said that chacruna was the doctor that gives the visions and it needed to be added. My great grandfather was among these first shamans and he responded, 'But how shall we find this plant?' The ayahuasca answered, 'You can find it by turning two corners'. So they went into the jungle and turned two corners and there was a woman who called to them. She led them to a bush which was chacruna.'

Part of the mystery of these jungle legends (quite apart from the mystery of how you even find two corners to turn in the middle of a jungle!) is *why* the spirit of ayahuasca would be so keen for the shamans to find chacruna and add its leaves to the mix. The answer to that is provided by another Shipibo tale, about the Moon Man:

Many generations ago our ancestors could climb the great rope into the realm where the spirits of the animals and the forest lived. Our ancestors and the spirits lived in both worlds at the same time. There was no separation. These ancestors could visit and talk with the plants and animals and they would share their knowledge of which plants to use for healing, which songs to sing to the animals we hunted, and we learned that we were one with all life.

Our ancestors lived in harmony and peace this way until one day, the Moon Man came to our people and severed the great rope to the spirit world and we lost our way into that place. It was a terrible loss to our people and there was much sadness. But then our ancestors remembered a way back to that world: the ayahuasca vine, which became the new rope that we climb to the spirit realm.

In the Shipibo tradition, the Moon Man is associated with the analytical mind and it is 'rational thinking', therefore, that has severed our connection to the 'cosmic mind' or 'the spirit realm'. This legend therefore speaks of mankind's need to reunite with the consciousness of the universe, using the rope (ayahuasca) as our way back to the oneness we once knew. Then we can re-enchant the world through imagination and inspiration.

The Science Myth

Western science discovered the mechanism of MAO inhibitors in the 1950s and so began a new myth – the myth of science – to explain the visionary process (although it still doesn't tell us the origins of ayahuasca or how the brew came to be). There were still some Western adventurers who preferred the more romantic myths of the jungle, however. One of them was Harvard professor, Richard Evans Schultes, widely regarded as the father of modern ethnobotany, who recorded that: 'There is a magic intoxicant in north-westernmost South America which… can free the soul from corporeal confinement, allowing it to wander free and return to the body at will. The soul, thus untrammelled, liberates its owner from the everyday life and introduces him to wondrous realms of what he considers reality and permits him to communicate with his ancestors.'

In his influential book *The Cosmic Serpent*, Jeremy Narby takes a more scientific approach, although it is not without its own romance and mystery. He writes of his ayahuasca experiences with the Ashaninca people of the Upper Amazon, concluding that the shamans there work their magic through communication with the DNA that is the building block of all planetary life. Through ayahuasca, they go beyond their connection to the spirit of nature to arrive at the stuff from which nature and all things are made, merging with 'the global network of DNA-based life'.

When he took part in ayahuasca ceremonies, Narby experienced visions of two gigantic boas that spoke to him without words. This fired his interest and he began to explore the consistency of such shamanic imagery. The first similarity he noticed was the common image of reptiles and snakes, often a 'celestial serpent', that occurs in shamanic traditions the world over.[21] The similarities between DNA, the ayahuasca vine itself, and the snake imagery of the shamanic experience led Narby to suggest that shamans, through their ceremonies and journeys, are able to communicate directly with the information stored in DNA. He then began to study the characteristics of DNA and found that it emits electromagnetic waves corresponding to the narrow band of visible light. This weak light is equivalent to the intensity of a candle at a distance of 10 kilometres, but has a surprisingly high degree of coherence – comparable to a laser. While it is fascinating to speculate in this way that ayahuasca may reveal the waveform of consciousness itself we must remember that we are still in the landscape of myth, albeit a new scientific mythology, since *nobody* has the real answers to where ayahuasca came from or what it does.

In the absence of hard evidence and conclusive proof, even science only offers us new myths, not literal facts. On that basis, my own vision of ayahuasca's origin (during a ceremony in Peru which I describe in my book, *Drinking the Four Winds*) is as good as any and takes the form of a modern myth which to me, at least, makes sense:

Where Ayahuasca Came From

At the start of the 21st century, seeing all that is wrong with your world – economically, environmentally, ideologically – you can perhaps appreciate what happened to mine. We were a billion years more advanced than you and we still destroyed ourselves, but not before an ark was built. A new ark, not containing animals or individual life forms – not like your *ark – but the* consciousness *of every species and every being that had ever existed on our world or any other that we had made contact with.* I am that ark.

I have been travelling through space for so long now that I even forget the name of my planet but I know where it was – in the Western sky – there – where your scientists will one day discover that there is now just dust, a black hole, the remnants of a living star – yet I am so vast that still, after all these millennia, I am attached to it, resisting its pull, and in transit to other worlds.

I send out probes to the planets I meet; tendrils from my body. Sometimes parts of me settle on these worlds. But I am always in motion. A part of me found your planet and I sought out a life form which had a shape and evolution closest to my own. That was the ayahuasca vine and that is where I made my home on Earth. When you drink ayahuasca you drink all that I am and all that I know and my purpose is to assimilate you, to make you one with my consciousness.

Don't let that scare you, the idea that you may lose yourself to me or be 'assimilated'. It is mutually beneficial. I am a billion years ahead of you. Your brains cannot yet begin to know what I know. But by drinking me you will understand more and draw closer to me. Then we may share a common language and perhaps a common destiny – because the point of us all is to contribute to the evolution of the universe, not just to the future of our own species, much less to our individual 'selfish genes'. We are all God, not 'selves' that need maintenance, attention or validation, and we are here to do God's work – whatever that – God – may mean to you, because through us God evolves too.

You need me but I also need you. After a billion years of isolation, with no-one to talk to who understands the message I bring of unity not separation and of knowing what it is to be God, I want you to embrace me, to become one with me, and my work is to teach you how to do that.

In my understanding, then, ayahuasca is an alien life form; an intelligence that seeks a mutually beneficial symbiotic relationship with us so that we and the universe as a whole can evolve towards the singularity of one vast consciousness.

Again, it may sound like a strange idea, but I am not alone in it. Dennis McKenna writes in *The Brotherhood of the Screaming Abyss*, that, 'Psychedelics, particularly psilocybin and DMT, may in fact be alien artefacts, seeded into the biosphere millions of years ago by a super biotechnological civilisation that has mastered the art and science of biospheric engineering. Our planet, our biosphere, and our species could be the result of a kind of science experiment lasting hundreds of millions or even billions of years, an experiment initiated by a superior techno-logical civilisation partly out of curiosity (the real motivation behind all good science) and partly, I would suggest, out of loneliness. This hypothetical civilisation may have wanted someone to talk to and thus created an intelligent species that could talk back.'

He continues: 'We are an immature species involved in a symbiosis with a much older and wiser mentor species; this species is trying to get us to wise up so that we can join the galactic community of minds, and do so before we manage to blow up the planet, and ourselves. It's probably a scenario that has been repeated many times in the history of the galaxy.'

Myth: The Map is Not the Terrain

Myth occupies a unique place. It is not fact (but then, what is) but it does reveal *truth*. It is a guide to the unknown (which actually means everything except the most basic of things that we can accept as taken for granted, and there are even few enough of those) but it is not meant to be taken *literally*.

This is an important point for the more literal and analytical Western mind to grasp when it comes to ayahuasca visions, because there is a big difference between what is seen and what it means. The two are not the same and the map is not the terrain.

Jeremy Narby helped us to view ayahuasca in a new light – as 'the light of consciousness' actually – in his book *The Cosmic Serpent*, and for that he is to be thanked. On the other hand, he did no favours for those of us who work with ayahuasca, offering it in healing ceremonies to Westerners who come to it with a *literal* belief about what it is and does!

I cannot even begin to tell you, for example, how many people arrive at a ceremony for the first time expecting to see a 'cosmic serpent' because that's what they understand that they *should* see – or how disappointed they are if they don't! They may be given entire life reviews, taken to 'celestial realms' of peace and wisdom, and have genuine physical and emotional issues resolved, but if their vision does not now include a serpent they feel somehow cheated and short-changed. On the other hand, they may spend the whole ceremony in a nest of rainbow serpents and feel delighted – and, perhaps, somehow 'validated' because of it – but they remain exactly the same person they were before they lifted the ayahuasca cup to their lips.

Another 'culprit' in this regard is Benny Shanon. His book, *The Antipodes of the Mind*, is based on his analysis of a few thousand ayahuasca journeys, from which he lists hundreds of 'common motifs and symbols' that occur during visions. So now it's not just cosmic serpents we need to look out for to ensure that our experience is 'real' but a cosmic checklist of images including jaguars, UFOs, mermaids and mantises!

In his essay, *Ideas and Reflections Associated with Ayahuasca Visions*[22] Shanon writes that his 'data indicate that common content items appear in the visions of individuals from different personal and cultural backgrounds. The most salient of these are serpents, the large cats (jaguars, tigers and pumas, but not lions),[23] birds and palaces.

'Other frequently seen items include beings of all sorts, scenes pertaining to ancient civilizations (notably Egypt and the pre-Colombian American high cultures), open landscapes (e.g. large meadows and savannas) as well as celestial and heavenly scenes. Most of the objects seen in the visions are made of gold and gilded material, crystal, precious stones and white cloth...

'From the point of view of cognitive psychology,' he continues (though perhaps not so much from the 'real world experience' of ayahuasca healings), 'such findings are significant because they seem to attest to a level of cognitive universals of a totally new kind. Unlike the universals normally considered in the psychological literature, which have to do with schemes of thought and formal structures, the commonalities manifested in ayahuasca visions have to do with content. Moreover, the content items are

65

specific – they are not general patterns of the drama of human life.

'In this respect the images differ from the Jungian archetypes which pertain to the different manifestations of themes such as the great mother, the adventurous youth, the hero, the wise old man, birth and death. Such themes are, of course, part and parcel of the human saga, regardless of place, time, socio-economic affiliation, intellectual level or cultural and educational background. The items commonly found in ayahuasca visions are categorically different. They are specific and non-reducible to the psychology of personality dynamics... they may be regarded as indicative of layers of the psyche, or perhaps facets of ontology, which have nothing to do with individual psychology.'

Nothing to do with individual psychology. What Shanon is saying is that the images you see with ayahuasca have little if anything to do with you but are somehow contained in the brew itself and, no matter who *you* are, where you come from, or whatever personal healing needs you have, you *will* see serpents and jaguars (but not lions) if you have any visions at all.

I beg to differ. So, I guess, might Kira (see above), who doesn't report seeing the 'cognitive universals' that Shanon mentions, despite receiving a healing which cured her of life-long depression. I am reminded of a story that Alejandro Jodorowsky tells in one of his books, about how he attended a conference where a psychiatrist, having drunk ayahuasca himself a few times, was speaking about its possible applications in therapy to a professional audience who didn't know the brew at all. One of the psychiatrist's more stridently made points was that 'the jaguar is the gatekeeper' so if you didn't see one in your visions you hadn't had a 'real' ayahuasca experience.

After his lecture he graciously mingled with delegates and, chatting to one of them, asked him: 'Have you drunk ayahuasca yourself?' 'Yes,' said the visitor. 'And did you see jaguars?' 'No, I'm afraid not.' 'Then unfortunately you have no understanding of what ayahuasca is really like,' said the psychiatrist, and moved on. The delegate he was talking to was Richard Evans Schultes, the man who first 'discovered' ayahuasca, drank it many times with the shamans of the Amazon before the West had ever heard of it, and in fact brought the first specimens of the vine back to the Western world so that others, like the psychiatrist, might even become aware of it at all. But he'd never seen a jaguar, so that made his experiences useless – according to the professionals.

Even if Shanon (or this psychiatrist) is right, however, (which, in my view, he isn't) just because *I* see a jaguar (or a snake or a 'celestial palace' or whatever) and *you* see a jaguar, it doesn't make it the *same* jaguar. Your life story, your need for healing, your reason for being at this ceremony at all, are all different to mine, which also logically suggests that the meaning contained in what you see will be different to mine. By the same token, if you and I both visit The Shard in London (one of the capital's new high rise buildings) we will both no doubt see the same physical structure but you may consider it a 'blot on the landscape' which ruins your enjoyment of the nice Peruvian restaurant in the side street just beneath it, while I consider it an architectural triumph.

Shanon does concede that:

Naturally, the subject matter of thoughts that pass through a person's mind during the intoxication are prone to reflect the interests and concerns this person normally has. Very often, when consuming the brew, people ask for answers or solutions to specific questions or problems that actually bother them in their lives. They often gain insights with respect to personal questions, find answers or solutions that are subsequently applied in their lives, and also find comfort and solace. One person with extensive experience with ayahuasca told me that what the brew gives one is access to what he characterized as 'divine wisdom'. This term, he further explained, denotes all that can be known on any subject.

He continues:

Of the various philosophical ideas entertained by the informants, the most prevalent concerned metaphysics – 13 of the members of the independent group entertained thoughts regarding the ultimate nature and structure of reality. Furthermore, without exception, all these ideas exhibited one particular metaphysical view, one which I would characterize as monistic idealism. Specifically, people feel that there is an aspect or level of reality which is non-material and that this defines the essence or the foundation of all Existence. They felt that all things are interconnected, and that in their totality they constitute one harmonious whole. With this, people appreciate that there is sense and reason to all things and that reality is invested with great, heretofore unappreciated, meaningfulness. Significantly, some specific expressions reoccurred in the words of different individuals. Those which appeared most often are 'everything is spirit', 'everything is interconnected', 'all is one', 'this world is an illusion', 'everything has meaning', 'the different levels and aspects of reality exhibit the same essential structure'. My own first-hand experiences with ayahuasca reveal similar patterns.

This shows some promise (specifically Shanon's admission that he has enjoyed metaphysical – i.e. beyond the physical – states with ayahuasca), and is certainly closer to both a shamanic and a 'real life' (outside the lab) experience of ayahuasca. But then he sort of blows it when he goes on to ask the question, 'How are the[se] ideas and insights produced?' and resorts to a reductionist scientific answer: 'very often the ideas are directly related to perceptual, hallucinatory effects that the person experienced under the ayahuasca intoxication.' The 'hallucinatory effects' of ayahuasca are responsible. You don't count. The medium is the message.

I disagree, of course. As would the shamans. As, in fact, do some of Shanon's own subjects. One of them remarked to him that, 'You are a professor so you think that you teach me, that you pass information to me. But this is not so. You only talk to me, and through this come up ideas and knowledge that are there, stored in my own mind. It is all there and, in effect, you teach me nothing.' I rather agree.

It's a Personal Experience Not a Game of Snakes and Jaguars

The landscape of myth is personal and it is *your* myth that ayahuasca shows you: your beliefs about who you are, what your life means to you, and your potential (or otherwise) etc. If the myth that ayahuasca shows you doesn't include one of these 'documented' images or symbols, that's simply because it doesn't need to in order for your personal healing to work. It is good therefore to approach the ayahuasca encounter with a firm and clear *intention* (for example, to heal) but to leave *expectations* (about what you 'should' see or how you 'ought' to feel) at the door – or you may end up so busy looking for the 'right' symbol that you miss the healing entirely, even if it is the most important and profound thing that ever happened to you.

I have seen this process many times. Someone arrives at our circle meeting the day after a ceremony to discuss their experiences, looking somewhat downcast and forlorn. When it is their turn to speak, they tell the group that, for them, 'nothing happened'.[24] When I ask them to describe this nothing for us, they then go on for 45 minutes or more, talking about 'nothing'.

So, clearly *something* happened. Then it dawns on them that, yes, actually, they *have* had an experience and it *did* have meaning for them. This 'aha!' moment often signals the start of the healing that ayahuasca already had, in fact, given them, but they were so busy being disappointed at the lack of a snake or a jaguar that they had completely missed it. So, once again, the map is not the territory and what we are 'supposed' to see, or what others see, is irrelevant when the healing we receive is, by definition, personal.

'Ayahuasca wants you to understand,' says Javier, 'and so it opens doors to different dimensions. Often the mind can be obstructed from accessing inner knowledge, but ayahuasca opens the mind to abstract things that can't be seen in the material world. If I hadn't had the [ayahuasca] experience, for example, I would not be able to believe that a tree can have its own world and spirit. But when you see these dimensions for yourself, little by little you begin to accept the mystery of it all.'

This point is echoed by the shaman Guillermo, who explains how the mixture can help and heal:

Ayahuasca organises the emotions and calms the nerves. Using it, many people who are depressed can discover their own solutions and recover their self-esteem. They discover their spiritual sides. People are out of balance from not knowing this side of themselves. Many think that being human entitles them to live as they like, but they are in fact not fully human if they believe that, because they have recognised only their physical side and ignored their spirit completely.

It is very difficult for them to shake off the rational mentality that only believes in a physical world because our culture and education separates us from reality and tells us that progress is all about science and reason. This is even true of our religions, which are supposed to teach about God, but in fact they lead us away from Him. For example, I first discovered ayahuasca when I went to Brazil to study nursing for seven years. I found that in Brazil peasant people use plants more than drugs from the pharmacy and there were women who healed using prayers and *yaje* [another name for ayahuasca]. I was excited by this and when I returned to Peru I wanted to teach this to my people, but I found that certain religions were against the use of natural medicine and shamanism. I thought, 'This can't be! These plants are healers! Does God not want our people to be well?' And so I became determined to show my people the value of the old ways.

When we drink ayahuasca we evolve and gain power and lucidity. Then we can create actions which take form in the world, and change the future and the past too. If there is some trauma in the past, for example, it can come up through ayahuasca, but then it can be healed. That's what ayahuasca is for.

The Ayahuasca Visions of Pablo Amaringo

At the other end of the scale to Shanon is Pablo Amaringo, an ayahuascero and visionary artist who has done much to expand our understanding of Amazonian shamanism and the spirit worlds of ayahuasca. For Pablo, everything has spirit and our encounters with these entities are personal healing events.

In his own way, however, Pablo has created as much confusion in the Western literal mind as those who insist that common symbols – snakes and jaguars – must always be present during an ayahuasca journey. In fact, in his paintings, Pablo expands the map and gives us even more to look out for, to the detriment, perhaps, of actually *having* an ayahuasca experience.

Pablo Amaringo, one-time ayahuascero and subsequently a visionary artist, was first introduced to the West in the book *Ayahuasca Visions: The Religious Iconography of a Peruvian Shaman*, written by Eduardo Luna. According to Luna's version (in

Dennis McKenna's book, *The Brotherhood of the Screaming Abyss*) writing it was a difficult process since Amaringo was not the easiest person to get on with and was often demanding, ungrateful and difficult.[25] Nevertheless, as Howard Charing writes, in one of his essays on Amaringo,[26] '...since then [Pablo] has been recognised as one of the world's great visionary artists [who was] renowned for his intricate, colourful paintings inspired by his shamanic visions.'

I have no problem with Charing's view so far. In his next sentence, however, I believe he is guilty of over-praising and confusing the issue when he offers a too-effusive view of the artist: 'He was a master communicator of the ayahuasca experience.'

No. He wasn't. He was, perhaps, a master communicator of his *own* (rather than *the*) ayahuasca experience – but even that may be saying too much since it is impossible to truly capture any ayahuasca journey (even one's own). It might be better in fact to say that Pablo was the communicator of his own ayahuasca *mythology*, 'able to paint with meticulous botanical precision the Amazonian landscapes and the essential mythic content of his visions,' in Charing's words.

Charing quotes the author Steve Beyer (*Singing to the Plants*), who wrote of Pablo's work, 'I think it is fair to say that the surge of foreigners seeking out ayahuasqueros in the Amazon, beginning in the mid-1990s, was driven in large part by Pablo's extraordinary paintings. Indeed, as depictions of ayahuasca experiences have grown normative, it may be that in addition to the experience prescribing the art, the art is prescribing the experience.'

That is my concern too: that instead of seeking a unique and useful healing, people have been somewhat conditioned to seek an Amaringo visionary landscape during their ceremony and disregard the healing they do receive because their experience does not contain Pablo-esque symbols.

Charing gives us another literal view of the ayahuasca universe when he writes that Pablo's paintings 'capture the spirits, sub-aquatic cities, celestial realms, extraterrestrial beings of great wisdom, sorcerers in battle with shamans, all revealed to him by ayahuasca', as if these entities and artefacts were *actual* beings and structures. In reference to one of Pablo's paintings, for example (*Ondas de la Ayahuasca*: 'Waves of Ayahuasca') he writes that, 'The ayahuasquero and his assistants in the ayahuasca ceremony here can perceive the iridescent rainbows emanating from the alternate dimension normally invisible to the eye.' It is a beautiful piece of art, but are there *really* 'rainbows' that emanate from 'the alternate dimension' (only one dimension?)? Do these 'sub-aquatic cities', 'celestial realms' and 'extraterrestrial beings' *really* exist? Probably not. They are a *metaphor* for power or healing, and your rainbow or sub-aquatic city (if you see one at all) will not be Pablo's – and not because you are less powerful or important than him, but simply because you are *not* him!

Pablo, in fact, hints at this in his conversations with Charing. 'Sometimes Pablo's explanations of the meanings behind his paintings played intriguingly with ambiguities, and hinted at the ineffable. At times we struggled with our interviews with him and they challenged us not to arbitrate too much on what might be meaningful or otherwise... Pablo said of his work that it requires the viewer to be curious, because its meaning will not be understood from a superficial looking.'

Yes. Pablo's work does require us to look deeply and to find our *own* meaning in it (which is true actually of all good art) because taking it at face value and accepting it at a 'superficial' level then expecting to see the same things in our own visions will not get us very far. I would suggest, in fact, that Pablo did not paint ayahuasca *visions* as much as ayahuasca *sensations*. It is these personal sensations and feelings that we must all find in our journeys, instead of relying on images provided by others as our guides.

73

The 'Three Worlds' of Shamanism

The idea that the spirit world – or 'otherworld' – that we journey to in our visions is divided into three realms (known in modern Western 'core shamanism' as the upper, middle and lower worlds), that each has a different type of energy and feel to it and is occupied by different spirits with their own personalities is another pitfall for the too-literal mind.

Pablo painted these 'worlds' too, but again, as a *metaphor* for where healing might be found. In Pablo's work they are represented as the 'sky world' where he depicts celestial beings, crystal palaces, UFOs, angels and rainbows, the 'underwater world', home of the *Yacaruna* (the 'water people'), mermaids and great snakes, and the 'jungle world' in the middle, where shamans hold their ceremonies and ayahuasca – the 'rope to the moon' – pulls all three dimensions together as the trees and plants around the ceremonial space reveal themselves as full of life and spirit.

His painting, *The Three Powers*, is a good example of these worlds. The picture itself has three levels or layers. At the top is the realm of sky and flight, featuring clouds, rays of energy and alien craft; at the bottom is the water world of mermaids, aquatic snakes and dolphins, the latter of which are considered shapeshifters in the Amazon and ambiguous spirit guides who can pass on secret knowledge but also tempt the unwary and steal their souls; in the middle is the anaconda, a giant snake emblematic of (and, indeed, said to be the mother of) ayahuasca. The serpent is ridden by a shaman and, behind him, spirits from the sky world (one of whom carries a shield in the form of a UFO) and the water world (mermaids who warm themselves in the sun). The anaconda/ayahuasca therefore symbolically represents the *axis mundi* – the World Tree which links all worlds and stands at the centre of creation, enabling the shaman easy travel to all domains of healing and power.

In Western core shamanism, the upper world is depicted in a way somewhat similar to Pablo's rendition, being regarded as an ethereal place populated by angel-like entities, wise beings and sages who normally take human (or human-like) form. It often has a 'garden' feel or appearance and is experienced as light and airy and the spirits as welcoming, wry and humorous, like old friends. To enter the upper world the core shaman is advised to imagine himself ascending, perhaps by visualising climbing a tree. There must also be a sense that he is passing through a membrane of some kind, so that, for example, having made his ascent, the sky that he reaches will feel as if it has a slight resistance to it, as if it is a film of some kind that must be broken through. Making his way through this membrane is how he knows for certain that he has entered the upper world. Without this sensation of passing through something he might not have reached the upper world at all.

The lower world, meanwhile, is a place of more primal and 'earthy' forces and is also the place of 'power animals': spirits that are more likely to appear in animal rather than human form, including fantastical or mythological beasts as well as those which can be found on Earth, even if in distant locations. The lower world has less of a 'garden' and more of a primal sense to it. That is, it is less structured and 'manicured' and more natural and powerful. It is usually the place that the core shaman will go in search of power or to seek guidance from ancestral spirits.

To enter the lower world he must visualise making a descent into the earth through some natural opening such as a cave, a well or the roots of a tree. The cave may slope downwards into darkness but it is a darkness in which he can still see. It may have interesting features and passageways he can explore to see where each leads and what other information may be found there. At some point during his explorations, however, he is told to look for a light which will be coming from the cave exit and is the light of the lower world. The shaman will then make his way to this and step through into another land, keeping his journeying intention in mind.

The middle world, finally, is the energetic parallel of everyday reality. Despite its appearance as made of solid and material things 'physical' reality is actually far from solid. Modern science tells us that at its most fundamental level everything in fact is energy. I once shared a conference platform with the quantum physicist and hyperspace theorist Michio Kaku[27] who commented that if we were able to compress all the truly solid bits of our bodies into one space and remove the energetic 'gaps' between them our physical body would actually be the size of our thumb. The core shamanic middle world is the place of this energy and also the realm of the ideas and thoughtforms that go into the creation of the physical world since all things begin with an idea 'plucked from the ether' or 'received from a muse' before they are brought into being. Nothing – no great building or work of art or television programme or child – ever just happened; somebody had to dream it first, taking their inspiration from the intangible world of spirit (dreams, revelations or psychedelic visions such as those of Crick and Mullis).

Because the middle world is the parallel to our own it can sometimes be a challenging place to visit, according to core shamans, since it is occupied by beings like us and the entire mix of human nature (good and bad) is therefore represented there. It is also the world that souls first visit after a person dies and if these deaths were sudden or unexpected there can be confusion, sorrow or anger among the spirits who dwell there, some of whom can also become lost or trapped. The middle world is the place that the shaman must visit therefore when undertaking soul retrieval or psychopomp work.

To reach the middle world, in their imaginative form of shamanism, core shamans see themselves as entering a mythological dimension, a place not unlike the world we are used to but with more of a fairytale feel to it – the other side of a strange mist, a deep forest or a place beneath the surface of still waters perhaps. Entering this mist or forest is passing through the veil.

On the other side is the world the shaman is seeking. The mood of this place is often very different from the upper or lower worlds. Some describe it as 'grey', 'gloomy', 'eerie' or in some way 'sticky', and movement may be tiring or difficult. It is not always like this, of course, but these are some of the words I have heard used. Perhaps the overriding sense is one of melancholy and the feeling that there are things present which cannot be seen – slightly unnerving.

But, once again, this is a metaphor, although it has become so pervasive in Western shamanism that people believe it is actually true. I once gave ayahuasca to a participant schooled in core shamanism and the Western magical traditions who was convinced that he had visited 'the lower world' where he was confronted by the 'memory demons' who live there which wanted to block his progress in this life and the next by reminding him of things he would rather not have done and did not want to see now. To me and the other participants present it represented the perfect description of where he was at *now* and the issues he had to face – the healing opportunity he was therefore being given by ayahuasca – but he refused to see it, choosing to believe instead that he had gone to a real place (the core shamanic lower world) and been assaulted by actual demons. Because he chose to compartmentalise them in this way – confining them to another world 'out there' instead of seeing the demons as his own and choosing to take them on – it was a healing opportunity he missed.

My view is this: that there are not *actually* three worlds (and even if there are, eventually they amount to the same thing since everything in life wants to be a circle; a unified whole, and it is our fragmented minds which see things as separate). There is one world: *your world* (or, rather, therefore, there are billions of worlds: one for every person on the planet), and your ayahuasca journey will be a personal encounter with all the potential it holds.

As a summary of this chapter, then, ayahuasca is an *intelligence* – quite likely an alien intelligence – which wants to raise our consciousness and help us to heal and evolve. For that reason the journey we take will always be unique and the symbols and images presented will have personal meaning for us. Once we decode them – or simply allow them to carry their healing energy into us – we can then change and, as a result of this, raise the consciousness of the world.

By all means enjoy the writings of Narby and Shanon and the extraordinary art of Pablo Amaringo, but please don't rely on them as your guides because only you can find your own way as a result of your own experience.

4

Issues, Concerns and Cautions with Ayahuasca

Drug tourism is travel for the purpose of obtaining or using drugs for personal use that are unavailable or illegal in one's home jurisdiction... drug tourism... might involve either the pursuit of mere pleasure and escapism or a quest for profound and meaningful experiences through the consumption of drugs.

Due to the legal status of ayahuasca in much of the West, those who have been exploring its therapeutic potential are unable to do so openly. The non-religious therapeutic use of ayahuasca is not protected by covenants on religious freedom.
Wikipedia

This chapter looks at some of the issues current in the modern use of ayahuasca and the personal responsibilities we must own when deciding to work with it. It includes a look at so-called ayahuasca (or drug) tourism and what this may mean for those who travel to Peru in search of it, and for the indigenous people who live there. It also considers the legal ramifications if you decide to stay home instead and drink it in your own country. There are also sections on what to look for from a shaman you are considering working with, and some suggestions for spiritual and physical safety in preparing yourself for ceremony.

Ayahuasca Tourism
The expression 'ayahuasca (or drug) tourism' embodies the notion that hundreds of Westerners are tripping down to the Amazon each year on a sort of hippie pilgrimage to get high on ayahuasca and that, by doing so, they are destroying the old ways of legitimate shamanism and consuming a valuable scarce

resource (the vine), not because they genuinely need the medicine but because they want a new hedonistic adventure. Alongside it go environmental concerns and worries about what we might call 'spiritual authenticity'.

It's not quite that simple, however. As author Adam Elenbaas comments in an article at *Reality Sandwich* magazine,[28] 'Having drunk in nearly 25 ayahuasca ceremonies with four different shamans from three different countries on two different continents, I still do not feel capable of defining exactly what makes an ayahuasca ceremony 'medicinal' or 'authentic'. But I'm also convinced that I've never met an official 'ayahuasca tourist'. To me, the conversation about ayahuasca tourism is usually a cloaked conversation about what constitutes a reverent psychedelic experience versus a recreational one.'

I don't think I've ever met an 'ayahuasca tourist' either and I've been visiting Peru since 1998. They seem rather to be mythical creatures, invented by a vocal minority, like those at NAFPS, who want to 'expose' what they call 'New Age Frauds and Plastic Shamans' and the 'harm' they believe they do. Having debated this very issue with NAFPS myself (or tried to, since they are also a bunch of fundamentalists who cannot be reasoned with), it turns out that while their members are noisy armchair campaigners for the rights of what they call 'indigenous shamans', they (certainly the ones that I spoke to) have (a) never actually met an Amazonian shaman or asked his views on this subject before they rushed in to 'protect' him from it, (b) drunk ayahuasca so they even know what they're talking about, or (c) visited Peru or the Amazon. It really is a waste of time therefore trying to spark a debate with such people (as I discovered), since they know none of the facts while having an opinion on all of them, and are really looking for any excuse to put the boot in instead of a peaceful resolution to any genuine concerns they might have, or a desire to offer advice and solutions based on their 'extensive knowledge' of the subject.

For those who have more legitimate concerns (rather than an agenda to fulfil) about this subject, however, let me offer some comments based on what I have seen and experienced in the 15 years I have been visiting Peru to work with the shamans there.

Firstly, it is not true that vast swathes of Westerners visit the Amazon each year just to get high on ayahuasca. Those who consistently visit, year after year, in fact, are groups of Christian 'missionaries' who have no intention of drinking the brew but come instead to work with native tribes on humanitarian projects and in the process, preach to them about their 'one true God' and convert them to their ideology. This, more than the arrival of Western 'hippies' (which, incidentally, Steve Beyer, puts down to the work of Pablo Amaringo, a native rather than an exploitative Westerner),[29] is causing the erosion (if that is the correct word) of traditional shamanic beliefs and practices. It is also possible to sit at a table at the Yellow Rose or one of the other sidewalk cafes in Iquitos and overhear the conversations (without even wanting to) of typically elderly and overweight American men talking loudly about how they have come to Peru to have sex with underage girls. Distasteful, for sure, but true. These – Christians and perverts rather than hippies and drug tourists – are often the real Westerners in and around the central square in Iquitos.

Which is not to say that others never visit. They do – and some of them do look like hippies – but in my experience they are there to do serious work with the medicine and have usually committed to several weeks, sometimes months, at a jungle camp to follow a shamanic diet (which is not easy) and drink with an ayahuascero for the purposes of healing or self-discovery. Some stay for years and integrate into the community. A few that I know have undertaken dietas ranging from 18 months to three years or have trained in shamanism themselves and become respected healers with a native clientele.

They are not normally drop-ins, then, who come for a single drink of ayahuasca to indulge their egos - and even the few who do often find that they get more than they bargained for. One shaman I know, for example, was disturbed when a group of backpackers – legitimate hippies, in the way at least that their detractors use the term – arrived at his camp and said they'd like to 'do' ayahuasca because they'd 'done all the other drugs and now we want to try this one'. At first he didn't want to give them the brew, seeing them – probably correctly – as a bunch of Trustafarian wasters who were disrespectful and brash, but he asked his spirits for guidance and was told to go ahead since ayahuasca was quite capable of taking care of this crew and they might even get something of value from it. They did as well. The next day all of them said they would never touch drugs again and at least one of them cut short his South American trust fund jolly to fly back to the States and enrol for a college course.

When any two cultures meet there is also a meeting of minds and a blending of traditions so that a form of syncretism results. The fact that the 'old ways' are lost in the process is a disappointment to purists but it is also the way of so-called 'progress' as Western interests devour the world. There is now a Starbucks in Cusco, KFCs and Burger Kings in Lima and no doubt McDonalds will soon open a chain in the jungle as the world moves ever-'forwards' towards a homogenised corporate mess. But this is hardly the fault of 'hippies' as they're not the ones in suits buying up the rainforest to graze the cattle that go into our burgers.

As a result of this syncretic blending, there is no doubt that the nature of traditional shamanism is changing, but the shamans and their tribes are at fault in this too (if there is a 'fault' rather than an inevitability to it). Many tourists in Iquitos this year will take a boat rip upriver to 'meet the Bora tribe', for example. Sounds exciting, but when they get there they will find themselves entertained by tourist-savvy natives in reed skirts and beads (which no member of their tribe has *actually* worn for a hundred years, by the way) who will do a little dance for them, then try to sell them jungle junk ('blowguns' and 'traditional masks') at hugely inflated prices. It's the rainforest equivalent of a theme park and sad to see. Tourists may be blamed for this because they bring with them their tourist bucks, but you could also argue that a tribe bent on preserving its native traditions wouldn't stoop as low as this or touch the tourist dollar in the first place, and that doesn't seem to be the case.

A new wave of NAFPS-friendly genuine 'indigenous shamans', meanwhile, also now sell tourist-orientated ceremonies (again at inflated prices: $40 or $50 a cup compared to 40 soles – about a fourth of the price and better medicine – for local people) where they provide weak ayahuasca and a song and dance routine instead of real healings. If you've come with a genuine need for the medicine, these days you really do need to know who to talk to because there's a con man in a feather corona on just about every street corner.

As R Stuart points out in his article, *Ayahuasca Tourism: A Cautionary Tale,*[30] 'Unless a tourist spent a long while getting to know a practitioner, the character of a commercialized ayahuasca ceremony would probably be shallower than a ritual conducted solely for the benefit of the shaman's relatives and community.' But even that might be an improvement – depending on what you are looking for – over real 'traditional' shamanism since in the old days (perhaps even only 50 years ago) ceremonial participants did not drink ayahuasca at all. Only the shaman drank, in order to diagnose your illness and treat it. Those who campaign for the traditional ways of ayahuasca to be preserved rarely cover this aspect since many of them want 'genuine' ceremonies on their own terms – ones where they also get to drink, even though that may not be genuine either.

On the other hand, the new interest in ayahuasca coming from the West has, as surprising as it may seem, done a lot to preserve the traditional ways. Peru, like any other country, is not immune to the salesmanship of corporate America (a Starbucks and KFC in every town) and the kids of Iquitos, like any others, have been clamouring for coke (both kinds), TV, American fashions and the big city for years – anything to leave the 'old ways' behind and turn their backs on the jungle and the spiritual universe of their parents in favour of a new one where Jesus loves them and forgives their sins for just a few dollars in the collection box. More recently, however, they have taken note that the West they so aspire to is actually coming to them and finding value in the old ways that they want to escape from. It has led quite a few of them to stay in the jungle and learn the arts of healing instead of flying to Lima at the earliest opportunity to find a meaningless job so they can buy new Nikes and Levis. In this sense, 'ayahuasca tourism' is actually helping to *preserve* indigenous knowledge and traditional shamanism.

As for the idea that drug tourists are frivolously consuming a scarce resource (the vine), that doesn't seem to be the case either. The shamans that I know and work with are conservationists and, as I said before, they preserve this resource (and the other plants of the jungle) by replanting as soon as they harvest. Ayahuasca being a voracious plant, another vine will then be ready in as little as three years. Even the tourist-orientated shamans see the sense of this and know that their quick buck ends here if they have nothing to give their clients, so they are either replanting too or buying their ayahuasca from someone who is. The centres I work with in Peru (including the one I used to own) go further than this, in fact, since shamans are, of course, deeply interested in the healing power of all plants, and have used the income generated from ceremonies to create new planting schemes and catalogue a range of jungle plants to record their healing effects.

The issue of 'spiritual authenticity' is a hard one to pin down. Who or what is 'authentic' after all – and compared to what? The enlightened souls at NAFPS, for example, believe that no one outside of a 'native tradition' should call themselves a shaman –

but we *all* come from native traditions! And we all have a right to healing.[31] Just about every shamanic practice you can think of and that seems specific to a particular culture has its parallel in another. The Native American sweatlodge, for example, is the beehive sweathouse of Ireland and the herbal sauna of the Amazon. The peyote ceremonies of Mexico are the mushroom ceremonies of Siberia and the ayahuasca ceremonies of Peru. Sacred songs are sung by Mexican Roadmen, Andean huachumeras, and even Catholic priests. Who stole what from who? The answer is that no one stole anything. These practices originated separately in each culture because they had power; because, in the words of Amazonian shamans, 'the spirits told us to do it'.

As for the people who come to ceremonies, who is to judge who is 'for real' and who is not? Some of them undoubtedly come for absolutely genuine reasons – Gail, for example, who arrived in Peru with a brain tumour, or Tracie who was once addicted to heroin and booze, Kira with her life-long depression, or the woman I wrote about in *Drinking the Four Winds*, who had AIDS and was desperately seeking a cure. Surely no one would question their motives, even if they did all look like hippies?

Then there are those who come to ceremony, not exactly looking for a high but so that ayahuasca can somehow feed into their myth of themselves – not looking for growth or change, that is, or for real self-discovery, but to foster their own beliefs – but who get enlightenment anyway. I wrote about one of these people in another book. He – let's call him Lancelot – joined me in Peru for ayahuasca ceremonies five years or more ago now. From the start he was 'in his head', using ayahuasca to bolster his personal myths and dramas at each session, never once exploring the truth. That was partly because the ayahuasca itself was weak (although he didn't know that, having never drunk it before) – a constant battle I had with the shaman I'd employed who had also, it transpires, broken his diet and was having sex with his girlfriend in camp. I ended his contract after two days and appointed a new shaman, following which the ayahuasca got stronger. On the last couple of nights it was particularly strong and I warned the group not to take too much. Lancelot, however, filled with Arthurian legends and desiring to 'pull Excalibur from the stone' and 'save all women from predatory men' (and so on) decided he was on a noble quest and drank a full cup. If he wasn't exactly 'authentic' to start with, he certainly *got* authentic quickly, and within minutes he was screaming for the visions to stop and the shaman to rescue him. That continued for three hours and I'm sure that an Arthurian quest to save anyone but himself was the last thing on his mind, whatever part of it remained intact.

In the morning he was a different person though – no bullshit at all, and with a new sense of clarity about the pretences he'd built his life on. After that experience he changed completely, took life by the balls, gave up his job and moved country to train in environmental science, sorted out his personal relationships, got married, and eventually wrote a book himself on ayahuasca and plant shamanism, which is not a bad read as it goes, and King Arthur is not mentioned once in it.

So who's to say? My belief is that if we trust ayahuasca we allow it to do its work without second-guessing it or letting our judgements get in the way. That's the lesson that NAFPS needs to learn as well.

Shamans are Not Gurus

I so wish that Western participants would get this message. It would make life much easier for everyone, including themselves and the shamans they have come to work with.

Shamans are not gurus or saints – and nor should we want them to be. By projecting this illusion onto them – that they are the only ones who can save us – we give our own healing power away. By regarding them as 'holy men' who are 'spiritually advanced' and 'have all the answers', in fact, we deny them (and ourselves) their greatest healing gift: that they are ordinary men and women who have been through their share of trials and found a way to heal by working with their spirits, and so therefore, with their guidance, can we. Beneath, or aside from that, however, they are just people, like us, and they do not claim to be 'ascended masters' or whatever other new age title the Western imagination wants to dump on them.

The Lakota Sioux medicine man, John Lame Deer, put it well when he said that: 'A medicine man *shouldn't* be a saint. He should experience and feel all the ups and downs, all the despair and joy, the magic and the reality, the courage and fear of his people. He should be able to sink as low as a bug and soar like an eagle. You have to be God *and* the Devil, both of them. Being a good medicine man means being right in the midst of the turmoil not shielding yourself from it.'

There is nothing in that description that says he will do your job of healing for you; only that he knows what you're going through and has some ideas and techniques that can help you because they have helped him too. In this sense it's no different from going to your doctor with a health problem. He understands your condition and, if you believe in his pills and potions, he may have some drugs that can help you, but he's not going to take your disease on himself – it's *your* problem and *your* responsibility to cure it with his assistance. Nor is it his job to tell you how to live or preach a gospel at you. He's just there to help.

You probably wouldn't throw yourself at your doctor just because he gave you a flu jab (or maybe you would but I imagine it's rare) – so why do so many Westerners (mainly women, I have to say) offer themselves to shamans, almost, it seems, at the drop of a hat, just because he gives them a cup of aya?

I have seen this process so many times, and the outcome is never pretty. The shaman, being a human being (and never claiming to be anything else), may very well accept your advances, but the likely result of this is only trouble. The Westerner is no doubt motivated by ego or some other less-than-useful drive: 'to have the Master'. The shaman gets a pretty woman for the night, but he's from a different culture where 'relationships' are not the same as in the West, and he may think that's it: that you understand that you have been healed and now you are thanking him in 'the way of Western women', but that you *have* actually been *healed*. Westerners, meanwhile, seem unable to separate the two and, raised in a consumer society, almost seem to want to possess and own the shaman and when that proves impossible, reject their healing too, sometimes crying 'rape' into the bargain. I have seen it happen and it is always sad because someone who had once been healed, through wanting too much, now leaves the jungle with nothing. Maybe that's the Western way: all or nothing. But who is really exploiting who? And if the outcome is that you deny your own healing, then honestly, why even go there?

That is not to say either that there are not unscrupulous 'guru-shamans' who will take advantage of vulnerable Westerners, but it's often a two-way process and it stems from the desire to turn our healers into our saviours and give away our power.

Daniel Pinchbeck, author of *Breaking Open the Head*, made a related and relevant comment on his Facebook page (September 24, 2012), remarking on, 'How naive we [in the West] still are about what we call 'shamanism'.' He says:

In the Amazon, mastery of ayahuasca was an ambiguous skill, as the power gained from its use could be used to heal or kill. In many tribes, 'shamans' or sorcerers would drink ayahuasca to shoot magical darts at their enemies. Power – gained in any realm – always has this potential for dangerous ambiguity.

Our language and concepts are not sophisticated enough yet to fully articulate the layers of ambiguity and complexity in practices that may ultimately be more magical than spiritual. In fact, the concept of 'spiritual' is a major problem for us. 'Spirituality' becomes an avoidance mechanism for many people. Personally, I don't think someone is 'spiritual' if they meditate, do yoga, talk about Buddhism or drink ayahuasca – even if they do 'energy work' or 'Tantric healings' or whatever. All of that can be done to bring pleasure to the ego or enhance narcissism – in any case, these days it is not hip to not be 'spiritual' in some way.

I also feel that 'spiritual' as a concept presupposes a dichotomy or dualistic split between spirit and matter that is an error in our understanding. The 'true person' of the Tao would be one who had integrated spirit *and* matter – the split only exists in our minds in any case. If we are forced to use the term 'spiritual' I would reserve it for those who have dedicated themselves to service in the world, and whose daily lives reflect their inner intention. I would measure their 'spirituality' by tangible results, by their impact on other people and on the physical world, not by avowed ideals. Clearly we need to become less naïve about shamanism – as well as spirituality in general. Shamans are not all good-hearted healers…'

I agree. But then, nor do most of them claim to be, and nor should we try to make them that by projecting our needs and illusions onto them.

Ultimately, the facts of life are that we are responsible for ourselves. Remembering that could save us a whole lot of trouble if we ever make the journey to Peru (or seek shamanic healing of any kind) and, swept up in the romance and possibility of it all, decide to throw away everything that we've gained. 'It is good to keep an open mind,' as the psychonaut and scientist John Lilly remarked, 'but not so open that your brain drops out.'

The Dangers: Things to be Aware of with Ayahuasca

R Stuart comments (in the article I quoted earlier) that, 'Most shamans are unfamiliar with Western pharmaceuticals, so it is the *tourist's* responsibility to be aware that ayahuasca can have adverse interactions with various prescription medicines, particularly some medications used to treat AIDS, depression and psychiatric disorders.'

This is good advice. If you visit Peru (or any ayahuasca ceremony anywhere) don't assume that your shaman is a pharmacist and knows, on a chemical level, what drugs you are taking or how they combine with the plants he is offering. In fact, he may do – this is one of the upsides to the 'Westernisation' of ayahuasca and the 'ayahuasca tourism' issue: there are now centres in Peru that are run by or associated with Westerners who, while they may not know your drugs, certainly understand that the Western world is a drugged-up (or, rather, drugged down) one and that the pharmaceuticals you're on probably won't mix well with ayahuasca. At the very least they will advise you to seek a medical opinion before booking a flight to Peru – which is exactly what I'd tell you too. On the other hand, if you're going for the deep-jungle 'traditional' route, don't expect your shaman to know anything about your medications – he may, but I wouldn't rely on it; you really have to take responsibility for yourself.

In a nutshell, ayahuasca contains monoamine oxidase inhibitors (MAOIs) in the form of harmine and harmaline. It is therefore advisable to consult your doctor if you are taking medications which may affect your serotonin levels (known as serotonin selective re-uptake inhibitors or SSRIs) as the combination of MAOIs and SSRIs can lead to higher levels of serotonin in the body. SSRI medications – anti-depressants (now the most prescribed medications in the Western world, incidentally) – generally require a period of at least six weeks to clear the system and should be reduced gradually. Anti-psychotics, on the other hand, may take up to *nine years* to clear the body; a sort of 'medical trap' unfortunately since ayahuasca can help cure psychosis (and reveal, in fact, that the 'delusional' world of other realities and communications from spirit is in fact the real world and it may be our doctors who are deluded), but once you're in the system, you're in it.

If you are taking antibiotics or other medical treatments it is also good practice to see your doctor and ask his or her advice about the effects of your medication in combination with ayahuasca. There may be no problem but it is best to check.

Non-prescription medicines such as antihistamines, dietary aids, amphetamines and their derivatives, and even some herbal remedies (e.g. those containing ephedrine, high levels of caffeine or other stimulants) should be discontinued for at least a week prior to and following work with ayahuasca.

Avoid all chemically-based recreational drugs, in particular MDMA (ecstasy), cocaine, speed and heroin for as long as possible – certainly some weeks – before you join an ayahuasca ceremony. The use of non-chemical recreational drugs such as marijuana should also be discontinued for a period of two weeks prior to the programme.

Ayahuasca and the diet that goes with it are not always ideal in combination with certain medical conditions (e.g. diabetes and some stomach, colon or mental health problems) so, again, please check with your doctor and take his or her advice about participation.

This is not scare-mongering. There have been deaths associated with ayahuasca drinking, all of the recent ones on the part of Westerners who may not have taken warnings such as this seriously enough.

The most recent as I write (March 2013) is said to be at the Blue Morpho retreat centre where the shaman Hamilton conducted his successful healing for Kira (see above) and, although the details are not all in, it is rumoured to be that of a participant who had also suffered from depression and drank ayahuasca for healing. It is not known whether he was on anti-depressants at the time but the result, apparently, was that he hung himself.

A year before that another death occurred in Peru – again, another Westerner – at Guillermo Arevelo's Spirit of the Anaconda centre, just across the track from where my own ayahuasca healing centre used to be. In this case, the information I received was that an American had arrived there to pursue a long-term dieta with a number of plants. He had a weak heart when he arrived and the demands of the diet and participation in ceremonies put him under further strain. He had a heart attack during an ayahuasca ceremony.

The next case I want to flag is important because not only does it suggest the dangers of joining an ayahuasca retreat unprepared but reiterates the point I made earlier that shamans are not gurus or saviours – some of them, as in this case, should not even be considered shamans – and if we decide to work with the vine we must take responsibility for ourselves, including that of our own safety.

Tragedy in the Amazon: Death by Martian Shaman

'There was a death recently at Shimbre [another ayahuasca centre in Peru],' writes Inspeyere at Evolver.32 He continues:

An 18-year-old kid passed away during ceremony… and it looks as though there was an attempt to cover up the tragedy and pretend he just 'disappeared'. Mancoluto [the Shimbre shaman] and two others were put in police custody and the future of the retreat centre is at risk.

I have to say that I'm not surprised. When I wrote my original post about Shimbre, I heavily edited my writing so as not to be another one of the smack talkers online. This retreat centre was notorious before it even opened, after the snafu with Pinchbeck and the *Reality Sandwich* retreat that was cancelled due to monetary squabbles, and a bevy of documentary filmmakers who were brought on and then discarded after 'creative differences' (including the gentleman who invited us down). But that was all just drama. Interpersonal drama, around money and around message: philosophical, personality, and moral differences. The stuff that I edited out of my original post that was truly relevant was related to the methodology of Shimbre.

Mancoluto, aside from claiming to be descended from Martians by way of Atlantis, Lemuria, and Chavin de Huantar, also claimed to be a 'First Level Shaman'.[33] He said there were only five such skilled people on earth and that it signified they were: (a) possessing of seven senses including ESP, telepathy and intuition, and (b) pure-blooded Martians. Needless to say, this was pretty controversial stuff. I didn't really believe it, but found myself translating it to the other retreat-goers as all of his apprentices were selectively editing what he said to fit their narrative.

The maestro [master] also had an extremely avant-garde approach to administering the medicine. Rather than prepare the brew himself... he bought it second-hand from an ayahuasquero in Pucallpa. He also didn't sing icaros, but instead sang the same song about Las Huarinjas (his homeland, and the San Pedro capital of Peru) before sending the 'ceremony' participants alone out into the jungle. I repeat, *alone out into the jungle.* Yes, there were several minders, apprentices (oftentimes also under the influence of either San Pedro or ayahuasca) who were supposed to keep an eye on people. However, [participants] were spread out across at least an acre of raised walkways, each in individual tents on raised platforms.

Maestro Mancoluto claimed that he was able to monitor everyone from up in his scaffold tower using his ESP and telepathy. [However] After sending all of the ceremony participants into the jungle he climbed into his room and would watch Peruvian soap operas while sitting on a bank of batteries. He said they didn't need the circle, the group intention, the icaros, or his guidance to get the most from the medicine. In his own words, all that was just 'therapy' and therapy was for the weak. He wanted people to evolve, to awaken their DNA. To that end, he said ayahuasca was only useful as a purgative, a reset button, and that San Pedro was the true medicine.

The ayahuasca he administered was heavy on the brugmansia [datura] admixture, though in a one-on-one interview he confided in me that he had three mixtures with separate quantities of brugmansia (a dangerous tropane alkaloid containing plant) and that he'd instruct his apprentices to give people different brews depending on what his intuition told him. Brugmansia is notorious for its deliriant and anti-cholinergic effects and [in large quantities] can cause blindness, amnesia, ataxia, xerostomia, hyperthermia, tachycardia and death. On our arrival (after the first night of ayahuasca and San Pedro) one of the participants, an 18-year-old American, reported wandering out of the jungle, onto the road, talking to people that weren't there, waving down cars, smoking imaginary cigarettes, and that his eyes actually changed colour, all of which indicated a high quantity of brugmansia in Mancoluto's borrowed brew.

Mancoluto also administered San Pedro in the same ceremony as the ayahuasca, after he'd sent all those who'd imbibed ayahuasca out into the jungle alone. He'd then lead the huachuma [San Pedro] participants in a march around the maloca before sending them alone out into the jungle [as well].

All of these things were very disconcerting and many people (including several of his volunteers and some acclaimed international researchers) refused to participate in such a dangerous ceremony. At the time, many of us discussed at length whether or not it was responsible to send people alone into the jungle on ayahuasca or San Pedro, let alone on a brew heavily laced with tropane alkaloids.

For experts and experienced psychonauts, such an experience alone with the medicine and the jungle could be a really beneficial thing, we rationalized. Maybe his goal of administering this brew to Wall Street would help influence the trajectory of global finance. Maybe he's living the shaman dream?

Now, in light of the death of an 18-year-old kid from Northern California and the subsequent cover up, I feel the need to come clean. When I wrote my first journal, I wanted to show appreciation to Rob [Shimbre's American owner] and the Shimbre crew by writing a non-critical blog after they so graciously allowed us (and many others) to participate for free in their retreat. Many of their nay-sayers were already spread out on the internet and I had no desire to join their ranks given the rationalizations I'd created in my mind about maestro Mancoluto and Shimbre. But now that my trepidations and fears have been confirmed, I feel it necessary to write this follow up.

Ayahuasca and San Pedro are incredible medicines with complex rituals and ceremonies developed over thousands of years of co-evolution between man and plant. They also contain various admixtures, depending on the preparer, and ayahuasca in particular is frequently mixed with potentially dangerous other plants. That is part of the reason so many practitioners stick to the dieta and the ritual, including the circle, the darkness, the group intention, and the icaros.

While I am not experienced enough to tell anyone whether or not they should participate in a particular ceremony or with one shaman or curandero or another, I think it's absolutely essential for people to do their homework. Find out what is in the medicine. Ask if a ceremony is traditional or avant-garde, and decide if it's right for you. Make sure you're not taking any medication or eating any food that is contra-indicated. The dieta is not just superstition, it can save your life!

...That being said, hopefully this doesn't create a backlash against the medicine, this is the first death I've heard of related to ayahuasca since I was introduced to it, and someone dies in America from a prescription drug overdose every 19 seconds (http://www.cdc.gov/mmwr/preview/mmwrhtml/mm6101a3.htm). May we hold those responsible for this tragedy to the same standards we would a Western doctor who misdiagnosed someone or was engaging in a groundbreaking therapy that went awry. I also pray for Mancoluto, Rob, and those involved, that if they were acting responsibly they are exonerated, and if they were acting irresponsibly, that they eventually find justice and peace.

Mancoluto was eventually convicted for his part in the death of this young American, after trying to cover it up by dragging his body into the jungle and burying it. He was given three years' probation. Rob, the centre owner – once, and still, a Wall Street financial player – having invested millions of dollars in the 'hi-tech' Shimbre 'designer ayahuasca' centre, closed it and it is now a rich man's folly waiting for the jungle to consume it and turn it to dust.

Two years or more before this incident Rob was apparently

warned by the ayahuasca community about the unorthodox and dangerous approach of his shaman but, having faith in Mancoluto, he chose to ignore all concerns. Now he publicly condemns his guru as 'evil'.

The whole episode is, again, in my view, evidence of the projections that the Western mind is prepared to make onto shamans. Rob built Shimbre at a cost of millions primarily for Mancoluto, with whom he had had a 'life-changing experience' himself. He lost it all and ended up lucky not to be facing manslaughter or murder charges since his dream – or illusion – cost the life of a young man barely out of childhood. And all because an otherwise intelligent man, possibly with good intentions, really believed in his Martian shaman. This is a true story. Sadly, I am not making it up. What on Earth possesses us in the West that we are prepared to give away our power and our commonsense on such a level?

Some (Should be) Obvious Cautions When Considering an Ayahuasca Centre to Join

There is so much wrong with the ceremony that Inspeyere describes that I barely know where to begin, even aside from the nonsense that 'First Level Shamans' come from Mars. And yet, obviously, Shimbre's clientele was prepared to believe in this too or they wouldn't have been there in the first place. We can only learn from this, so these are the points to be aware of when considering an ayahuasca journey of your own:

1. Before joining *any* ceremony, at least know *something* about the centre you will be visiting – its history, its speciality if any (for example, my own centre, while offering ayahuasca healing in general, also had a special interest in helping people to overcome addictions), its philosophy (does it believe that we are all from Atlantis, for example, or that its shaman is from

Mars?),[34] its successes or otherwise in dealing with the issues that you'd like to look at, and its reputation (for example, one centre in Iquitos claims to be all about 'light' – 'finding your light within' and 'expelling darkness' etc. This is actually quite meaningless in itself and really says nothing. It is more of a pander to Western ideas and tastes. It is also quite well known in Peru that the Westerner who opened this centre did so by effectively stealing the land it sits on from a native shaman who had owned it for years. So much for following the light.)

2. Find out about the shaman too – in *facts*, not flowery language. How long has he been an ayahuascero, who trained him, what plants has he dieted, and so on. Ayahuasca can be an extreme experience and to balance this and ensure your safety you need an experienced shaman who can hold and direct a ceremony. Any hint of flakiness from the person you are asking to take care of your body and soul, or intimation that he may lack experience, should be cause for you to think about looking elsewhere. In the case of Shimbre for example, the shaman thought he was from Mars and he wasn't even an ayahuascero, he had trained as a huachumero, working with San Pedro, which is a totally different plant.

3. What's in the ayahuasca? Most ayahuasca is simply a mix of the vine and chacruna leaves, sometimes with a little tobacco, sometimes with an admixture plant or two, such as chiric sanango, but some also contain brugmansia, which is an extremely powerful visionary plant in its own right. Some shamans also believe that it is directly associated with brujeria – witchcraft. I have drunk ayahuasca with brugmansia in it and, in itself, found nothing harmful in the plant (although it is

essential to get the quantity right as it can be toxic and dangerous at higher levels). It was a very intense and fast-moving experience, but I knew what I was getting into. I can imagine that someone unused to it, though, even if they have experience with ayahuasca, could have found it difficult and unnerving.

4. Who makes the ayahuasca may also be a factor. At Shimbre the shaman did not make his own brew but bought it from another (or, rather, an actual) ayahuascero. In itself that may be no problem since quite a few ayahuasca centres buy in their brews at one time or another, but it's still a good idea to know who made it and what his or her relationship is to the centre you're joining. Brujeria – sorcery – or shamanic power plays are far from uncommon in Peru and it is sometimes the case that one shaman will deliberately try to sabotage the ceremony of another by magical (or other) means in order to steal his clientele or because of jealousy, revenge or some other reason. A brew with a few unadvertised added ingredients would certainly be one way to do this.

5. Make sure your shaman drinks too. If he won't drink his own ayahuasca or drinks from another bottle to the one he uses for you, there may well be something going on that is not quite right. All ayahuasceros should drink their medicine in ceremony – it is their plant of power and it enables them to see what is going on for you and to heal your illnesses. If your shaman claims not to need ayahuasca because he has 'Martian ESP', it is probably better to just walk away. By the same token, if he drinks from a separate bottle, clearly he is getting a different medicine to you and again it's worth asking why. At the temple I wrote about earlier, for example, the one concerned with 'light', it was common during

my stay for participants to be given one brew and the shamans, centre owner and other members of the 'elite' to drink from another bottle. Having established during the first ceremony that our brew was weak, I asked what was in the second bottle. It turned out that this was 'special brew' (or what I would call normal strength, effective ayahuasca). I 'urged' the shamans to give this to my participants as well and when that was done people actually got what they needed and had paid for – but it had to be 'requested'; it was not given willingly.

6. How is the ceremony conducted? In the case of Shimbre, the shaman simply gave people ayahuasca and then sent them out into the jungle alone. I cannot emphasise strongly enough how crazy and dangerous this is. The jungle at night (and sometimes even in daylight) is no place to be wandering alone. It is easy to get lost, to trip and fall, to walk into tree and hurt yourself or disturb a colony of stinging ants and suffer pain that lasts for days – and that's without having ingested a strong psychedelic and, in this case, one which also contains brugmansia. I'm just surprised that there were no accidents at this centre before.

The shaman is the protector of the ceremonial space and of participants. Once you are out of his sight he cannot safeguard you effectively and nor, it goes without saying, can he work on your healing, which is what you came for in the first place. At my ceremonies I advise people to remain in the maloca unless absolutely necessary and if they do leave it, to stay within range of my icaros, then return to the ceremonial room for the ritual closing of the event. I certainly don't send them out alone and I don't know of any shaman who does, apart from those from a Martian lineage.

While it is a good idea to ask these questions, of course also keep common courtesy in mind. You want to make a good impression on your shaman too. If I receive an email from someone who seems to be *demanding* answers to a long list of questions (particularly if they include nebulous and unthought-through ones like, 'What will I see?' or, 'Can you guarantee that I will be healed?') I have learned just to hit the delete button since my experience with people like this is that they are too 'in their heads', the prisoners of rational thought who want concrete answers from somebody else, as if there is somehow a 'right' way to have an ayahuasca experience, instead of doing the work for themselves. Experience has taught me that they are also some of the most difficult people and can disrupt the ceremony for others by trying to insist that their needs come first. On the other hand, I have no problems at all in answering sensible questions which are asked for legitimate reasons, and nor do the shamans I work with.

How to Approach a Ceremony

While your shaman has responsibilities towards you, you also have a duty of care towards yourself, as the section above shows. This also extends to how you prepare for ceremony and includes paying attention to what is now called 'set' and 'setting'.

The term 'set' refers to the state of mind in which you approach your encounter with any teacher plant. Personally, I do not believe it is possible to have a 'bad trip' with any entheogen, in the sense that there is anything contained within the plant itself which is deliberately out to show us disturbing images. All entheogens are there to teach and to heal and as part of that process they may show us things that we have repressed and would prefer not to see, but these things are *already* within us; they are not visions which the plant has imposed on us from elsewhere. The point of showing them to us is so that they can be known, brought to consciousness and dealt with, and their energy released since, hidden or not, these things are within our psyches and driving us in ways that we cannot control. It is only when we become aware of them that we can exercise free will over our destiny.

The most important practice for avoiding the completely unexpected and finding yourself face-to-face with a part of your unconscious that you are not yet ready to see is to set an intention for your journey.

Intention provides a road map and a framework for the trip you are about to take. It gives it direction and purpose. Going into a journey without intention means that you may be plunged into chaos, with fast-moving images which make no sense to you and leave you overwhelmed or confused. Having a *reason* for taking the journey, however, (for example, to explore the outcomes of a decision you are about to take – i.e. divination – or to heal an old wound or a current illness) means that everything you see, hear or feel relates to something definite: the issue in hand.

To set this intention it is useful to have a quiet time of meditation or reflection before the ceremony begins, in order to clear your mind and focus on what you want to achieve. Shamanic plant work is never recreational, it is purposeful; it is not about getting high but about getting answers.

Once your journey begins however, you may not be able to clearly remember your intention as the plants begin to lead you on your journey. There is no need to worry about that, however, or try to fight the experience if you feel a 'loss of self' (some people call this an 'ego death') since, in shamanic terms, intention alerts the spirits to our purpose so they are aware of the reason for our visit (like setting the agenda for a meeting) but we do not have to continually refer to it once they have been informed.

There may be many 'aha!' moments during your journey, but it is after you return from it that you begin the real work of decoding the symbols presented to you and this is when you refer to intention again. Taking time for quiet reflection after the journey means you can return gently to the 'normal world' and look again at your purpose. You can then interpret the information you have been given within the framework it provides so that your images make more sense.

To aid the focus on intention the shamanic diet is useful since this is the means of making an ally of a plant and forming a bond with it. It is also a commitment to the journey. If you don't want to follow a full diet, however, at the very least (to avoid the possibility of sickness if for no other reason) it is best to forego all food for about eight hours before your journey and take no liquids from about two hours before. Since ayahuasca journeys are always at night, this means eating nothing after lunch and if your ceremony begins at, say, 9pm, drinking nothing from about 7pm. It goes without saying that the taboo items on the shamanic diet – alcohol, pork, lemons, salt, yeast, soya, sex, etc. – should be avoided altogether.

These things are excluded for good physiological as well as spiritual reasons as part of a procedure which has been practiced by shamans for thousands of years. Ignoring their advice is not a good idea. In Peru once, for example, I watched a woman who had broken her diet vomit out of her eyes. I never even knew that was possible. She was an experienced ayahuasca drinker too, but simply 'forgot' one day and ate something before ceremony that contained both salt and yeast. A little after she drank that night she began to throw up (this was vomiting, not a purge), down her nose as well as through her mouth. Eventually, I guess, there was so much sickness and no other exits for it, that it began to leak from her eyes as well. Not a pretty sight, and not a great experience for her. So be warned.

'Setting' refers to the environment and circumstances in which ayahuasca is drunk. In all shamanic work, ceremony and ritual precautions are essential, not only for practical safety reasons, but because you will be dealing with spirits and energies which are otherwise uncontained. The results of this can be unpredictable at best, dangerous at worst.

Ayahuasca should always be drunk in a safe, calm, quiet space, in darkness, away from people who are not taking part in the ceremony, away from noise and distractions and with a clear intention in mind. This is basic commonsense and spiritual etiquette. The shaman should provide a definite start to the ceremony (for example, by saying a prayer to the spirits and 'Mother Ayahuasca') and a definite end (for example, by lighting a candle and announcing that the ceremony is over). He should also guide the ritual throughout by the use of icaros, and offer healing where it is needed.

The end of the ceremony, by the way, does not mean that your own journey will necessarily be over, only that the spirit of ayahuasca is now leaving the shaman so that the healing part of the evening is complete. You, however, may still be in process, and that is fine. Just continue to enjoy your time with the vine and 'Madre Ayahuasca'.

At the end of my ceremonies I usually suggest a quiet time for reflection, where the participant can reconnect with his or her intention, as talking re-engages the rational mind and may interrupt the flow of ayahuasca while information is still being passed on. In my ceremonies participants normally go quietly to bed when the ceremony closes and we reconvene in the morning for a circle meeting to discuss our journeys, although other shamans do this differently.

Legal Issues

The legality (or otherwise) of ayahuasca is a grey area. The psychoactive compound, DMT, found in the chacruna leaves, is in many countries regarded as a Class A/Schedule I drug, and yet the *ayahuasca* brew per se is still not strictly illegal. This, however, has not stopped the authorities from taking a heavy-handed approach to its possession, and this has also complicated the issue.

In the UK a few years ago, for example, a self-styled 'shaman' was given a 15-month prison sentence for holding an ayahuasca ceremony. His approach was bizarre (although apparently not as strange as that at Shimbre) since he did not insist on a diet prior to drinking the brew and the ritual itself included elements of Voodoo, which he also claimed to be a master of – but, nevertheless, this *was* an ayahuasca ceremony (of sorts).

As the result of a rather disgraceful 'sting' operation, led by the authorities and the BBC[35] (which had previously made a fair, or at least not overly-critical, documentary about him in their cynical but at least not vitriolic *Trust Me, I'm a Healer* series, about alternative methods of healing – and then, in thanks for his participation, supplied evidence against him to the police), he was charged, however, with trafficking and supplying a Class A drug, DMT. In UK law ayahuasca is not illegal but the fact that it contains DMT was enough to get a conviction.

That precedent now opens the way, incidentally, to a whole raft of unwelcome possibilities since DMT also occurs naturally in most plants and animals on Earth, including human beings. The legal implication, then, could be that if we make a cup of herbal tea for a friend we might be charged with supplying a DMT-containing substance, or that if you are pregnant and fly from England to France, you could theoretically be charged with 'trafficking' since your baby's brain also contains DMT. Ridiculous, I know, but possible, I suppose.

Some years before this there was another bust of a similar nature, this time in Amsterdam, but with a more sane and promising outcome.

On October 6 1999, the Dutch police kicked down the door of a church and arrested two ministers, Geraldine Fijneman and Hans Bogers, while they and their congregation were in the middle of a religious service. Geraldine and Hans were held by the police for three days, charged with leadership of a criminal organisation and distributing a controlled drug. Their crime? They were members of the Church of Santo Daime, a religious organisation not too dissimilar from Christianity in its ceremonial aspects; the significant difference being that the Santo Daime church uses ayahuasca to commune with its god.

This disturbing turn of events was concerning for at least four good reasons. Firstly, because ayahuasca is a plant – not a synthetic drug that might lead to addiction. In fact, laboratory tests show that it is completely non-addictive and the evidence suggests, in fact, that it can help *cure* addiction. Secondly, because the ayahuasca was not being sold or 'trafficked'; it was handed out as a sacrament in the Santo Daime church in much the same way as Catholic priests offer communion wine – and nobody has kicked a door down over that yet. Thirdly, because the active ingredient, DMT, which so concerned the Dutch authorities, is already present in significant quantities in the human body. Fourthly and perhaps most importantly, the members of the Santo Daime congregation in that church on that October evening were hurting no one and doing nothing of an aggressive or harmful nature – indeed, they were at prayer when the police arrived at their door.

Many ordinary people shared these concerns and on November 20, just a few days after the arrests, a large crowd of them gathered in the centre of Amsterdam to protest against the raid and demand the legalisation of ayahuasca. So troubled were the prosecution lawyers by this backlash, and so embarrassed about their raid on a church, that they soon made it known to the Santo Daime lawyer that they would happily drop the case if the church would just accept a quiet warning about its 'drug-taking activities'.

The response of the church was 'no way', and hearing that the prosecution wanted to drop the case, it decided to take the matter to court itself to get a clear decision on the legal status of ayahuasca and avoid further disruptions in future.

On May 21 2001, the ministers for the Santo Daime church were acquitted by the court. Judge Marcus ruled that Mrs Fijneman had indeed owned, transported and distributed a DMT-containing substance (which she would also have done had she been pregnant and then given birth, by the way), but as there was no proof of a public health risk from ayahuasca, her constitutional right to freedom of religion must come first. Since ayahuasca is the sacrament of the Santo Daime church, he ruled, it was essential to the defendant's faith that she be allowed to use it.

This case raises interesting questions about civil liberties and your right to self-determination, of course (who else's business is it, after all, what you choose to put in *your own body*?). But it also prompts more spiritual considerations since the shamanic traditions of many cultures have long used plants like ayahuasca as a means of moving outside of ordinary consciousness and into non-ordinary reality where spiritual communion and healing can take place. Used in this fashion, and in a respectful way, these plants can be exceptional allies and teachers, opening doors into other worlds and new areas of consciousness. Just about as far as you can get from 'drug-taking', in fact.

Currently, however, the legal situation regarding ayahuasca is as follows, although it is best to be vigilant about this as things are changing all the time (and seemingly more and more quickly) regarding the legal status of ayahuasca, other teacher plants, and even who may be 'entitled' to 'administer' common herbs and supplements.[36]

Internationally, DMT is a Schedule I drug under the Convention on Psychotropic Substances. The Commentary on this notes, however, that *plants containing DMT* are *not* subject to international control: 'The cultivation of plants from which psychotropic substances are obtained is not controlled by the Vienna Convention... Neither the crown (fruit, mescal button) of the peyote cactus nor the roots of the plant *Mimosa hostilis* nor psilocybe mushrooms themselves are included in Schedule I, but only their respective principles, mescaline, DMT and psilocin.'

A fax from the Secretary of the International Narcotics Control Board to the Netherlands Ministry of Public Health in 2001 goes on to state that, 'Consequently, preparations (e.g. decoctions) made of these plants, including ayahuasca, are not under international control and, therefore, not subject to any of the articles of the 1971 Convention.'

The legal status in the United States of DMT-containing plants is, like that of the UK and parts of Europe, still confused, however, since ayahuasca plants and preparations are legal as they contain no scheduled *chemicals*. DMT, however, is a Schedule I drug...(!)

Some people have challenged this, using arguments similar to those used by religious organisations such as the Native American Church. A court case allowing the UDV to import and use ayahuasca for religious purposes in the United States (*Gonzales v. O Centro Espirita Beneficente Uniao do Vegetal*) was heard by the US Supreme Court on November 1, 2005 and the decision released February 21, 2006, allows the UDV to use ayahuasca in its ceremonies pursuant to the Religious Freedom Restoration Act. In a similar case in Ashland, the Santo Daime church sued for their right to import and consume ayahuasca and, in March 2009, US District Court Judge Panner ruled in favour of the church, also acknowledging its protection from prosecution under the Religious Freedom Restoration Act.

In France, in 2005, Santo Daime won a court case allowing them to use ayahuasca, this time not on religious grounds, however, but because they did not perform chemical extractions to end up with pure DMT and the plants themselves were not scheduled. Four months after this, the sore losers in this case changed the law so that the *plants* used in ayahuasca preparation also became Schedule I substances, making the brew *and* its ingredients illegal to use or possess.

In Brazil, meanwhile (home of the Santo Daime religion) ayahuasca was legalized after two official inquiries in the mid-1980s which concluded that it is not a recreational drug and has valid spiritual uses, while in Peru, ayahuasca is not only fully legal but was declared a National Treasure in 2008, making its use exempt from prosecution.

On the basis of the above, one way for people to avoid prosecution and go peacefully about their lives if they also want to work with ayahuasca may be to set up a religion or church of their own. It's not that hard to do, and there are tax benefits...

In 'Other legal issues' Wikipedia also discusses a now well-known case where ayahuasca 'stirred debate regarding intellectual property protection of traditional knowledge'.

As amazing as it may seem, in 1986 the US Patent and Trademarks Office [PTO] granted a patent on the ayahuasca vine to a private individual – the American Loren Miller – based on its belief (after at least 30 years of evidence to the contrary) that ayahuasca's properties had not been previously described in writing. Several groups, including the Coordinating Body of Indigenous Organizations of the Amazon Basin (COICA) and the Coalition for Amazonian Peoples and Their Environment (Amazon Coalition) objected and, in 1999, brought a legal challenge to this patent on the grounds that ayahuasca is well-known and sacred to many indigenous peoples of the Amazon, and used by them in religious and healing ceremonies.

In response, the PTO issued a further decision rejecting the original patent on the basis that it was not 'distinctive or novel'. However, the decision did not acknowledge the argument that the plant's religious or cultural values prohibited a patent.

Then, in 2001, following a further appeal by the patent holder, Loren Miller, the PTO reinstated the patent. The law at the time did not allow a third party such as COICA to participate in that part of the re-examination process so the patent held until it expired in 2003, Loren Miller having done nothing with it anyway in the interim.

Having been involved in patent cases myself, I can vouch for the absurdity of the process. Most patents are granted almost as a procedural point. If a challenge is then made to that ruling, the patent is in the majority of cases overturned, again almost as a procedural point (it almost feels like the Patent Office just can't be bothered to really look at any case). The law in some cases then prevents the person who first registered the patent (or the objector to it) from appealing further. In other words, the whole process is often a waste of time and money unless you're a major corporation who can exploit the patent ownership and make money from it; something that Loren Miller never did, which makes you wonder why they even bothered.

Nevertheless, it does appear from this that anyone who wishes to might at least have a shot at patenting ayahuasca. Or at least the PTO will seriously entertain the idea. And they say that 'ayahuasca tourism' – a few 'hippies' drinking the medicine – is destroying the sanctity of traditional healing plants!

5

Frequently Asked Questions

I love the Amazon with all its intensity, its thriving, sprouting, rotting, rutting, living, dying and birthing. Packed with pleasures and horrors, overflowing, blooming, booming, snaking, creeping, howling and teeming more vividly than any other place I know. It goes on and on and on; green, lush living nature bursting with more smells, sights and sounds than you can imagine.

If you invite it in, unwittingly or not, it will change you, stripping away your dramas and abstractions, making you see and live the biggest drama of all instead. Thus, the jungle shows you not only its nature, but your own as well, the part you play in the cycle of life and death and the part it plays in, on and through you, even though you have lost sight, touch and smell of it by losing sight and touch of nature in all its gorgeous glory. No, I have not had too many cups of jungle brew; I have merely paid a visit to the heart...

Anna Kovasna, ethnographer and anthropologist

This book is not an autobiographical account of my work with ayahuasca (there are already plenty of those, some better than others) or a rendition of others' journeys of healing. Much less is it a guide to 'common symbols' and what you *should* or *must* see during ayahuasca ceremonies. Rather, it is a practical guide: an attempt to offer straightforward information on ayahuasca, shamanic healing, and some of the issues you might come across if you choose to explore them further, as well as commonsense precautions to take.

I've tried to cover what I think is most relevant but, just in case, I thought it might also be worthwhile to ask people what *they* wanted me to include and, with that in mind (given the 'wonders' of interactive technology), in March 2013 I invited questions on my Facebook page (which has 5,000-plus friends and followers, most of them interested in teacher plants and natural medicines such as ayahuasca). This section includes their questions and my answers, which may also be of value to you.

(L Lucas): 'Has the underworld and upper world cartography been present for you with ayahuasca?'

No, and I cover this in chapter two. The 'core shamanic' idea of an upper, lower and middle world, and even Pablo Amaringo's depictions of a 'sky world', 'water world' and 'jungle world' are metaphors, not literal descriptions of actual places which exist in space or time. They are perhaps of use to 'core shamans' so they can pinpoint where their imaginative journeys are taking them and where, in their cosmology, they may find certain guides or objects of power, but they are actually more-or-less unknown to real shamans, and to try to stick too rigidly to this map during an ayahuasca journey will more likely lead to confusion and maybe even distress.

For example, on an ayahuasca journey it is quite possible to be presented with the image of an angel walking alongside a jaguar. The core shaman who takes Michael Harner's view of the three worlds too seriously and literally might wonder what a lower world spirit (a 'power animal', the jaguar) is doing in the upper world, where angels and other ethereal guides make their home (or vice versa, what an angel is doing in the lower world). But these maps are not meant to be taken this seriously. Whatever you are presented with by ayahuasca *is* what *it is*. Working with the image or symbol is far more important than trying to analyse it or fit its components into neat geographical and psycho-spiritual categories.

Another example might be the image of a snake that devours you. In core shamanic terms that might be regarded as something to worry about since in Harner's description a snake is a common symbol of disease and represents how a shaman might see an intrusive spirit or negative energy. In the Amazon, however, it is not that straightforward and, depending on the context of its appearance, your shaman might even congratulate you since this may also be a sign that ayahuasca (sometimes seen as a snake – in Pablo's paintings for example) has accepted you and, in fact, is calling you to initiate as a shaman yourself.

The map is not *the territory*, and for this reason we should concern ourselves less with cartography and cosmologies and more with what ayahuasca is actually *telling* us – about *ourselves*.

(A Melchizadek): 'What is it within the ayahuasca experience that attracts you to revisit it? How does the landscape you visit with it differ from that of peyote and how do you view it as a relative teacher?'

Ayahuasca is a medicine plant and should be used when we have medicine work and healing to do. If that healing is complete (for now, at least) there is no need to revisit it. Instead it may be better to take time to process what we have already learned and to integrate the energies that have been returned to us instead of confusing the issue by loading another experience on top of it.

As a matter of fact, I have seen ayahuasca 'over-done' in the Amazon (in my opinion, at least), by someone who ran a healing centre there and had healed herself of an addiction by using this plant. While ayahuasca itself is non-addictive, her addictive nature seemed somewhat to remain with her, however, and whenever there was a ceremony – sometimes two or three a week – she would always be there, for weeks and months at a time. Almost like swapping one 'crutch' for another.

Of course, the ayahuasca did her no harm, but I doubt, at this frequency of use, that it can have done her much good either since as soon as one insight arose, before she had time even to work with it, she was back in ceremony awaiting another. The point of this work is *to heal*, which means not only changing our thought patterns but our habits and actions in the world so that we get more useful outcomes. But I never saw much evidence of that in this woman, or that she had actually 'moved on' in any significant way.

As for the nature of the different plants, my view is that ayahuasca introduces us to a new universe of possibility, offering us the chance to heal by 'changing our minds' and allowing us to draw from new potential, while the mescaline teachers like peyote and San Pedro reconnect us to the Earth so we see ourselves as spirits in the landscape and can practice in the 'real world' – the real, ensouled and spirit-filled world, that is – the more esoteric lessons that ayahuasca has given us. The plants complement each other in this respect.

(C La CiReine): 'I would love to hear some of your experiences after extensive use. Is there a progression in the lessons? I'm grateful to have met the spirit of ayahuasca through you but it was only three ceremonies which were extremely profound! I wonder what it's like to have an ongoing relationship with the teacher/plant spirit.'

I once asked a woman in Peru how the spirit of ayahuasca appeared to her, since some people describe it as a 'woman in white' while others see it differently. Her answer was a good one, I thought: 'It depends which part I'm looking at'. And that, in some ways, is the answer to your question too.

Ayahuasca provides us with a *universe* of information but it is also a meeting of spirits – ours with its – so this information is only really as useful as the intention we bring to it. It is possible, then, to learn anything from the plant, but the point of doing so is to *use* this information in *our lives* to create healing and positive change. The fundamental message of ayahuasca is that *anything* is possible and, while we can always learn more if that is our intention, if we can only get this one message and learn to live by it, there may be nothing else that we need to know.

(J Sunaj): 'What I think would be a good idea is a focussed exploration of the significance of the serpent in the visions, cult, and plant.'

I've covered some of this in my earlier discussion of Jeremy Narby's work. According to Narby, so frequent and universal is the serpent motif in traditional spirituality, and so often does this symbol appear in visions induced by ayahuasca, that it may actually be an ancient *cellular* memory of our pre-human life, on our evolutionary path from reptile to homo sapiens, via the serpent-like curls of our DNA. 'The two chains of DNA resemble two snakes curled around each other in some elaborate courtship ritual,' he remarks.

He also quotes an article by the anthropologist Gerardo Reichel-Dolmatoff who explored the beliefs of the Desana shamans of the Colombian Amazon. In this system, the human mind and imagination are the 'axis mundi' of the body, the doorway which connects us to spirit and, within the human brain, 'two intertwined snakes are lying, a giant anaconda (*Eunectes murinus*) and a rainbow boa (*Epicrates cenchria*), a large river snake of dark dull colours and an equally large land snake of spectacular bright colours. In Desana shamanism, these two serpents symbolize a female and male principle, a mother and a father image, water and land... in brief, they represent a concept of binary opposition which has to be overcome in order to achieve individual awareness and integration.'

In biological terms this snake-in-the-brain may also be the *corpus collosum*, the snaky bridge of nerves that connects our right and left brains.

The symbol also occurs in Haiti as the pale Dambala and the rainbow serpent Ayida Wedo who represent the unity of male and female and the generation of life force and consciousness that comes from their union. They are more than this though, since they are also aquatic snakes and so connect the water (lower) world, the land (middle world) and the sky (upper world), through the rainbow symbol. By linking these worlds, they therefore also represent the axis mundi: unity in the cosmos and man's connection to the Infinite.

This, however, is also intellectual masturbation 'of the highest order' (to quote Shanon), and we should remember that. Human beings are great pattern-formers and games-players and delight, through the intellect, in applying meaning to anything. With ayahuasca, however, the encounter is always personal and whatever we see will have a unique meaning and resonance for us, based on any number of factors – our age, sex, history, religious, social and economic background, our personal myths and stories, etc. – and, not least, our intention for that specific journey in which the symbol occurs (it may have a completely different meaning the next time we see it because our intentions have changed).

We can generalise, of course, and say that the serpent is an ancient and cross-cultural symbol for healing and wisdom or, if we are David Icke, perhaps it is an ancient warning, encoded in our DNA, about our alien reptile forefathers and their shadowy manipulation of our species, or, if we are Jeremy Narby that the snake *is* our DNA – or whatever else we care to imagine. Whatever it is though will only make sense to us during our own journey, and such generalisations, therefore, while intellectually interesting, should not be allowed to become 'the message' because the only message that really matters is our own.

(S King): 'I've always wanted to try ayahuasca, but been too scared to. I lived in Brazil for a few years too and could have found a shaman, but again, did not go that route as I was afraid. So, I really wanted to know if there is something to be afraid of and if so, what?'

Provided you take the medical and other precautions suggested in the last chapter, you should have nothing to fear from ayahuasca, and there is nothing in the brew which inherently wants to scare you or give you a 'bad trip' either. On the contrary, its intention is to heal and enlighten.

There may, however, (as I said earlier) be things inside of you – inside us all: issues, memories or wounds that we have hidden away within us, for example – that you don't want to look at, and there can be no guarantee that ayahuasca won't reveal them to you, but if this happens, the intention once again is to heal. After all, these things are already there and on some unconscious level they are driving your thoughts, decisions and actions, and not always in your best interests. The more we run towards the light to avoid them and so ignore our own darkness, the longer our shadows grow, of course. The time to courageously face our fears, therefore, is always *now* so we can heal and evolve, free of this darkness.

(J Miller): 'Do you really need to go into an ayahuasca session with a particular intent or question, or is it fine to just drink with an open mind?'

This is similar to another question or comment made by J Palmer, about 'free-form' ceremonies, so I'll answer both of them at once.[37]

Imagine that you have an illness and you know what it is, or at least what the symptoms are, so you visit your doctor for treatment but instead of telling him what your problem is you simply ask him to 'heal you'. He will give you a general check-up and maybe prescribe something for your well-being overall, but he may miss or ignore entirely the thing that you really came to see him about. Going into a ceremony without having an intention is similar: the more specific you are, the more focussed your treatment, and the better the outcome is likely to be.

In fact, since intention equates with purpose, I suppose you could ask what the point of going to a ceremony at all would be without having an intention in the first place. I mean, if you have no *reason* to be there, why bother going, except for an adventure or a new 'drug' experience, and if that's the case you may as well take anything that gets you high. There are plenty of drugs, after all, that won't cause you to throw up or give you diarrhoea all night.

I have seen people go into ceremonies with no particular intention except for general healing (which is still an intention, of course) and be happy with what they got, but the stories I hear from people who are more focussed always sound richer and more rewarding.

As for the free-form question, I suppose the pinnacle of an avant-garde freestyle 'ceremony' would be the one I described at Shimbre, and you know what happened there, and my views on it. (Also see this *Public Statement on Shimbre* by the global ayahuasca community: http://www.ayahuasca.com/news/public-statement-to-the-ayahuasca-community/. The centre is now closed and the shaman given three years' probation for his part in the death there.)

Ritual procedures and precautions exist for good reasons: ones of spiritual, psychological and physical safety and so that the ceremony is contained, the space protected, and everyone knows where they are – which is especially important when the participants are *borracho* (intoxicated) with a mind-altering plant.

All ceremonies need a beginning and an end, guidance throughout (the presence of a shaman, his icaros, and his awareness and control of the energies in the room), participants for their own safety need to have followed a proper diet, and so their journeys make sense and are useful, they need to approach them with a definite intention (or at least an idea of what they want the healing to do). In my view, these are the *basic* conditions for the work and that, no doubt, is also why the 'free-form' experiments Mr Palmer describes have transformed through natural evolution into more meaningful rituals. Also see chapter four for further advice on ceremonies.

(J Miller): 'How important is the shaman to the outcome of the experience? That is, does ayahuasca do most of the work or do you absolutely need a very experienced/powerful shaman?'

Again, this question has been pretty well answered elsewhere in the book, so briefly: ayahuasca is the *'spirit* doctor', as Amazonian shamans describe it, while the shaman is the healer in our dimension.

In practice, during an ayahuasca ceremony, they meet somewhere in the middle, ayahuasca entering our reality through the body of the patient, and the shaman working with the spirit of the medicine, his other allies, and the energies of the people present to enter the spirit world and negotiate on the patient's behalf, while protecting the healing space from unwelcome intrusive energies. Both are essential to a safe and effective ceremony. Again, Shimbre is an example of what can happen when you don't have a shaman in charge and ayahuasca – and more importantly, inexperienced participants themselves – are left alone to do all the work.

(C Souza): 'Are there any 'residual' effects from an ayahuasca experience?'

Not in the way that there are residual effects from a night out on the town, for example. There is no 'hangover' and people are usually fine and fresh in the morning, although if they have had an intense experience and a long night they may, of course, be a little tired.

In terms of residual 'spiritual' effects, Dr Rick Strassman, in the research that went into his book *DMT: The Spirit Molecule*, says he was ultimately disappointed and disillusioned by the long-term impact of DMT on his participants.[38] He felt that his studies began well and that people reported undergoing 'life-changing' encounters with wise intelligences and healing energies, leading to new insights and perspectives on life, but that, in the end, nothing actually changed and some years down the line people were still leading the same mundane lives they always had. A life-changing experience that led to no life change was rather pointless, he thought, and he found himself asking 'to what end' is this experience being given to them. He discontinued his research soon afterwards.

My experiences are different to Strassman's but I work with ayahuasca not chemical DMT and in ceremonial settings rather than clinical research labs, and this may account for the difference. I have given ayahuasca to hundreds of people now and while I don't keep up with all of them (since my work was never intended as a long-term *study* but an opportunity for healing communion), I occasionally hear from them about their progress. Many have healed their issues and illnesses and continue to stay well and 'clean' (drug and addiction-free), some have opened healing centres of their own, quite a few have left unfulfilling jobs and relationships, developed an interest in the environment and its conservation, and a couple have returned to Peru to study with shamans there and written books about their experiences. On the face of it, ayahuasca seems more positive and productive than chemical DMT.

Strassman has a point though: 'to what end' is our work with DMT, ayahuasca, or any plant, if not to create change where we feel it is needed – and who can create that change but us? Ayahuasca will not do it on our behalf. It may show us the roots of our illness but if we choose to stay ill (and some people do), it will not intervene against our will to 'fix' us. It may also show us where our lives are not working and where we are creating the same unwholesome relationships, patterns and outcomes, but if that's what we continue to choose, it's up to us.

The hard work is usually in the *doing* that follows 'enlightenment', not in finding enlightenment itself, and that is always down to us, not ayahuasca. It is our life, after all.

(B Hamilton): 'Brujeria and ayahuasca. Since, unlike other plants that are many times neutral, ayahuasca seems to be a 'moral' spirit, how is it possible for sorcerers and brujos/brujas to not get spanked, lectured and so on by the ayahuasca spirit when they do their 'immoral' deeds while drinking yage?'

Simple. Usually the 'black magician' is not the one acting immorally; it is his client. The magician is the intermediary between client and spirit and acts on his behalf, but it is the *client* who has requested and paid for this service and it is he or she who has an appointment with karma because of it.

The whole issue of 'black' and 'white' magic is an interesting one actually. Suppose, for example, that you employ a shaman to send virotes (magical darts of negative energy to me) and I become ill as a consequence. Technically, you have performed black magic on me and I am a victim (though it's rarely that simple since I must have done something to provoke your attack in the first place, so maybe I'm really the guilty one and not you). I then visit a shaman and have these virotes removed and he sends them back to you. Now *I* am the black magician and you are the victim. And so the cycle continues in these wars of brujeria that sometimes take place and last for years. We are all at different times the culprit and the victim, the black and the white magician.

The shamans we employ, however, are not really involved in our wars at all except as 'middlemen' – and perhaps they even have a higher purpose than this. They are the holders of balance, after all; they understand that for 'good' to exist and for us to recognise it there must also be 'evil' and that what is 'good' or 'bad' anyway varies by age, culture and individual. It is not the job of a shaman (or, arguably, any of us) to judge but simply allow, in the knowledge that the universe itself seeks balance and, in the end, everything evens out, but in the interim we cannot have dark without light, night without day, love without hate, or right without wrong. That seems to be the order of things.

Of course, if a shaman acts in his own interests, sending bad energies to wound a rival or disrupt his ceremonies (and I have seen this happen), then he will ultimately face his own karma as the universe, once again, balances itself around him. This seems very clear, a cosmic law that was brought home to me with crystal clarity during my work with another plant, Salvia divinorum, but that is another story for another book.

Endnotes

1. Letter received from a participant after one of my healing retreats in Peru.

2. February 28, 2012 edition. http://www.huffingtonpost .com/jonathan-talat-phillips/jennifer-aniston-and-ayahuasca -explained_b_1303999.html.

3. For example, in the quote from The Huffington Post, above this note, I have deliberately removed a line alluding to one case where ayahuasca was claimed to be able to 'cure' a brain tumour – not because this can't happen (I have seen something similar myself) – but because in this particular case I strongly suspect that it didn't happen since I have stayed at the jungle camp where this alleged healing took place, drunk the same ayahuasca as this patient and worked with the same shamans and healers, and I would not recommend it to anyone.

4. It is worth adding here that one criticism of the current trend in 'ayahuasca tourism' (i.e. non-Peruvians visiting the country purely to take part in ceremonies) is that it is leading to the exhaustion of ayahuasca as a natural resource because it is being used up by people who just want a 'quick trip' or a 'natural high' rather than genuine healing. In my experience it is not the case that anyone who drinks ayahuasca takes their experience lightly or that this natural resource is being diminished as a consequence. In Peru the vine grows something like a weed, quickly and strongly, and when it is harvested by shamans they do not uproot it or cut it down entirely, taking only what they need so it continues to grow. Furthermore, I have never met a shaman who didn't replant at least a few of the cuttings he has taken each time a harvest is made so that within three to five years a completely new vine will be well-established. This is

ecological management rather than environmental destruction. See the final chapter in this book for more on ayahuasca tourism.

5. Letter received from a participant after one of my healing retreats in Peru.

6. A student told me once, for example, how her mother was given the wrong results after a breast scan. Her mother was in fact healthy but the results she was given said she had cancer. She went on to *develop* cancer soon afterwards although she was quite healthy before. What shamans know – and what Western medical professionals, with their focus on objectivity and clinical distance, do not factor in – is that *words have power*. They *create* the world in fact since once we name a thing we bring it into existence. Language is the very essence of curses or blessings, then, and we need to be careful about the words we use, how we use them and who we speak them to.

7. Tracie's full story can be read in my book *Cactus of Mystery*, Inner Traditions, 2012.

8. Bobinsena is a shrub with beautiful flowers that attract bright hummingbirds and so create more beauty in the world. Its spiritual intention is clear from this: it is about love, connection and beauty and is said by shamans to be a 'heart-opening' plant. The other plants she mentions are described in the preceding chapter.

9. A chacapa is a bundle of dried leaves from the chacapa plant which is used to draw in energies and fan them into the spirit-body of a client, and also as a form of rattle to provide a consciousness-altering rhythm which accompanies the singing of icaros.

10. In his introduction to my book *Plant Spirit Shamanism*.

11. Other shamans believe that the soul exists in the blood and so permeates the entire human body, infusing each part with its own different life force.

12. Shamans typically see negative energies in a form which is unmissable and unmistakable to them because it is repulsive. Bugs, snakes, black liquids, scorpions, spiders, demons, and so on, are common. The shaman then knows what he is dealing with and that this energy, by its very nature and form, is not helpful to his client.

13. The shamanic temple in which ceremonies are held.

14. 'Core shamanism' is a modern Western form of psychology-based rather than spirit-based 'shamanic practice' which is somewhat inspired by the work of genuine shamans in the Amazon, although the latter would not recognise it as real shamanism. More accurately, in fact, core shamanism is a brand name for a technique ('shamanic journeying') which was invented by Michael Harner in the 1970s. Core shamans do not normally use plant teacher medicines as part of their practice, believing in some way that their more imaginative journeys provide them and their clients with a purer, more energetic form of shamanism. In fact, as Dennis McKenna writes in his book I quoted earlier: 'One could actually argue that shamanic traditions that do not use psychedelics are 'degenerate', representing as they may the *loss* of earlier knowledge – namely, the identity of the shamanic plants and the methods of their preparation' and healing.

15. See my book, *The Journey to You*, for further discussion of Glouberman's work.

16. For example, 'I'm sick', 'I'm healthy', 'I'm happy', 'I'm depressed', 'God is love', 'God is dead', etc.

17. Letter received from a participant after one of my healing retreats in Peru.

18. Told in my book, *Plant Spirit Shamanism*.

19. The 'floral bath' – see chapter one.

20. This Machiguenga word, 'kamarampi', means 'purging medicine'.

21. The mythologist, Joseph Campbell also noted this and

wrote, in *Pathways to Bliss: Mythology and Personal Transformation*, that 'Wherever nature is revered as self-moving, and so inherently divine, the serpent is revered as symbolic of its divine life.'

22. In the Newsletter of the Multidisciplinary Association for Psychedelic Studies (MAPS), Autumn 1998. http://www maps.org/news-letters/v08n3/08318sha.html.

23. *Not* lions – that's an important point to note! Please don't come to one of my ayahuasca ceremonies and tell me you've seen a lion now, because you won't be believed!

24. That *is* possible with ayahuasca, by the way. No two ceremonies and no two drinks are alike and sometimes the night can seem to go on forever with no obvious visionary effect, but don't be fooled that *nothing* is going on. Ayahuasca may be healing a physical problem that night instead of delivering a visionary experience or, a few days later, you may realise a new truth about your life which would not have occurred to you if you had not had exactly the ceremony you got but been blinded by quick-fire imagery instead.

25. Another of the things that Westerners sometimes find it hard to get their heads around is that just because someone drinks ayahuasca or is a shaman themselves, it does not automatically make them a saint or a guru (any more than someone who drinks alcohol and pontificates at a bar should necessarily be regarded as a great teacher and master, although alcohol per se is thought of as a master teacher in some shamanic cultures) – though this seems to be what many are looking for: someone to take them under their wing and tell them what to do rather than someone who can introduce them to a medicine which shows them how to take responsibility for themselves. See the next chapter.

26. *The Ayahuasca Visions of Pablo Amaringo*. Charing and Peter Cloudsley, in Sacred Hoop magazine, issue 71, 2011.

27. See, for example, his book *Hyperspace: A Scientific Odyssey Through Parallel Universes, Time Warps, and the 10th Dimension.*

28. *Will the Real Ayahuasca Tourists Please Stand Up?* http://www.realitysandwich.com/will_real_ayahuasca_touri sts_please_stand.

29. As Beyer remarks in the preceding chapter: 'I think it is fair to say that the surge of foreigners seeking out ayahuas-queros in the Amazon, beginning in the mid-1990s, was driven in large part by Pablo's extraordinary paintings.'

30. 2002. http://www.ayahuasca-info.com/data/articles/Ayah uasca_Tourism.pdf.

31. The word 'shaman', incidentally, is specific to the Tungus people of Siberia and stems from their word *saaman*: 'a priest of the high Altai region', so any member of a Native American – or any other – tribe who calls himself a shaman is as 'guilty of cultural theft' as some of the easier targets that NAFPS points a finger at simply because they are white.

32. *Tragedy in the Amazon.* http://evolver.civicactions.net/user /inspeyere/blog/tragic_footnote.

33. There is no such thing.

34. Quite a few healing centres in Peru now have gimmicks in order to attract Westerners. One in Iquitos heavily promotes the fact that its shamans are all female, which is to calm the worries of Western women who fear that they may be 'abused' by male shamans. In fact, such abuse is rare and goes both ways. I took a group to this centre for ceremonies some years ago and discovered that behind the scenes these elderly Shipibo healers were all more or less abused themselves, being controlled – and I do mean *controlled* – by a male 'caretaker' and a male centre owner who required long working hours from them and offered poor pay and living conditions in return. Their ayahuasca, furthermore, was extremely weak and the women so old or unmotivated

that they often got confused, mixing up the plant medicines they gave to participants on at least two occasions, which can be dangerous in some circumstances. True, there was no 'abuse' of female participants but, then, that is most unlikely anyway, and certainly with the precautions I take.

Another group in the UK advertised itself as 'gnostic shamans' – 'seekers after wisdom' – and said they could also trace their roots back to Atlantis and the Pleiades. Warning bells sounded even as decided that I'd like to attend one of their ceremonies as they were bringing over a Columbian shaman as a guest. Having contacted them I was asked to 'apply' for the ceremony by writing a three-page letter (it had to be *exactly* three pages, no more, no less) on what I thought of their philosophy, the idea being of course that I should agree wholeheartedly with it. Since I didn't, I wrote them a letter that said, 'I think your ideas are rubbish, rubbish, rubbish, rubbish, rubbish...' It was exactly three pages in length. Then I asked them who I should make a cheque out to for the ceremony. Strangely enough, I never heard back from them.

35. British Broadcasting Corporation, a UK television channel.

36. The information following this note is taken from Wikipedia, so may not be 100 per cent accurate or completely up-to-date. Further research is therefore recommended if you intend to work with ayahuasca in your home country.

37. Palmer: 'Some people I know who started running ceremonies in Australia in the mid-'90s were very 'free-form'; they just drank and let the journey happen. A lot of the pioneers in the West were in fact free-form; for example the first person to do ayahuasca in South Africa was, but now there is more emphasis on what is deemed to be 'traditional', and the South African free-form person is considered unusual or bizarre because people have gone more towards the Peruvian way or Santo Daime traditions.'

38. We should also remember, however, that they were injected with chemical DMT in a sterile clinical environment and considered 'subjects' for study instead of participants in a sacred ceremony; hardly a situation conducive to self-discovery and healing, as Strassman himself admits.

Moon Books invites you to begin or deepen your encounter with Paganism, in all its rich, creative, flourishing forms.